LEARNING FROM KOHUT

Progress in Self Psychology
Volume 4

Progress in Self Psychology

Editor, Arnold Goldberg, M.D.

LEARNING FROM KOHUT

Progress in Self Psychology
Volume 4

Arnold Goldberg
editor

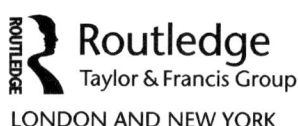

Routledge
Taylor & Francis Group

LONDON AND NEW YORK

First published 1988 by
Lawrence Erlbaum Associates, Inc., Publishers

This edition published 2012 by Routledge

2 Park Square, Milton Park, Abingdon, Oxfordshire OX14 4RN
52 Vanderbilt Avenue, New York, NY 10017

Routledge is an imprint of the Taylor & Francis Group,
an informa business

First issued in paperback 2020

ISBN 978-0-88163-081-7 (hbk)
ISBN 978-0-367-60649-7 (pbk)
ISSN 0079-7294

Contents

Contributors

Howard Bacal, Training Analyst and Former Director, Toronto Institute of Psychoanalysis; Associate Professor, Department of Psychiatry, University of Toronto.

Howard S. Baker, M.D., Clinical Assistant Professor of Psychiatry, University of Pennsylvania, Philadelphia; Attending Psychiatrist, Institute of Pennsylvania Hospital, Philadelphia.

Margaret N. Baker, Ph.D., Clinical Assistant Professor of Psychology, Hahnemann University, Philadelphia; private practice, Philadelphia.

Michael F. Basch, M.D., Professor of Psychiatry, Rush Medical College; Training and Supervising Analyst, Chicago Institute for Psychoanalysis.

Bernard Brandchaft, M.D., Training and Supervising Analyst, Los Angeles Psychoanalytic Institute; Assistant Clinical Professor of Psychiatry, UCLA School of Medicine.

Douglas W. Detrick, Ph.D., Director of Psychology Training, Adult Psychiatric Outpatient Clinic, Stanford University School of Medicine; Clinical Faculty, Psychiatry Department, University of California School of Medicine, San Francisco.

Barbara Fajardo, Ph.D., Director, Infant Follow-Up Research, Developmental Institute, Michael Reese Hospital, Chicago; Faculty, Doctor of Psychotherapy Program, Institute for Psychoanalysis, Chicago.

Robert M. Galatzer-Levy, M.D., Faculty, Chicago Institute for Psychoanalysis; Lecturer, Department of Psychiatry, University of Chicago.

Robert J. Leider, M.D., Training and Supervising Analyst, Chicago Institute for Psychoanalysis; Assistant Professor of Clinical Psychiatry, Northwestern University School of Medicine.

Sheldon J. Meyers, M.D., Training and Supervising Analyst, Chicago Institute for Psychoanalysis; Assistant Clinical Professor of Psychiatry, Pritzker School of Medicine, University of Chicago.

Jule P. Miller, Jr., M.D., Director, and Training and Supervising Analyst, St. Louis Psychoanalytic Institute; Clinical Assistant Professor of Psychiatry, St. Louis University School of Medicine.

Anna Ornstein, M.D., Professor of Child Psychiatry, University of Cincinnati College of Medicine; private practice of psychoanalysis, Cincinnati.

Carl T. Rotenberg, M.D., Fellow, American Academy of Psychoanalysis; Assistant Professor of Psychiatry, Yale University School of Medicine.

Estelle Shane, M.D., Founding President, Center for Early Education and College of Developmental Studies, Los Angeles; Visiting Lecturer, Department of Psychiatry, UCLA.

Morton Shane, M.D., Director of Education, Training and Supervising Analyst in Adult and Child, Los Angeles Psychoanalytic Society and Institute; Associate Clinical Professor, Department of Psychiatry, UCLA.

Marion F. Solomon, Ph.D., Coordinator of Mental Health Training Programs, Department of Continuing Education in Health Sciences, UCLA Extension; President, Continuing Education Seminars, UCLA.

Robert D. Stolorow, Ph.D., Member of the Faculty, Southern California Psychoanalytic Institute; coauthor, *Psychoanalytic Treatment: An Intersubjective Approach* (The Analytic Press).

David M. Terman, M.D., Training and Supervising Analyst, Chicago Institute for Psychoanalysis; Attending Psychiatrist, Michael Reese Hospital-Psychiatric and Psychosomatic Institute, Chicago.

Paul H. Tolpin, M.D., Training and Supervising Analyst, Chicago Institute for Psychoanalysis; Senior Attending Psychiatrist, Michael Reese Hospital, Chicago.

Ernest S. Wolf, M.D., Training and Supervising Analyst, Chicago Institute for Psychoanalysis; Assistant Professor of Psychiatry, Northwestern University Medical School.

Acknowledgment

The preparation of this book was financed by funds from the Harry and Hazel Cohen Research Fund. Ms. Chris Susman provided secretarial and editorial assistance.

Introduction

Douglas W. Detrick

As psychoanalytic self psychology has moved from infancy to toddlerhood, the annual self psychology conferences have fostered and borne witness to this developmental process. The papers and discussions from the early conferences were published under a variety of titles. Each of the volumes has also included work other than those presented at the highlighted conference. This volume is no exception to that tradition.

The first section comprises two papers describing the experience of being supervised by Heinz Kohut. It is of course most interesting to hear about the person whose genius it was that launched self psychology. These first-person accounts also offer specific clinical material presented personally to Kohut, enabling us to learn substantially more about how Kohut would handle particular clinical quandaries in a way not presented in any of his published work.

Section Two, Integration of Theories, is a treat for its readers. It presents the most current, "cutting-edge" contributions to psychoanalytic theoretical discourse. One could not find a more sophisticated presentation and discussion of the crucial theoretical issues facing contemporary psychoanalysis: Psychoanalysis has a long history of rejecting rather than attempting to integrate new ideas with its classical model. Dr. Stolorow and the Drs. Schane each break with this long tradition and attempt an integration, although their proposals follow "vastly different routes."

Robert Stolorow, the first contributor, continues his work urging that self psychology (and for that matter all of psychoanalysis) jettison any metapsychological pretensions and stick to a clinical, "experience-near" perspective. Another part of his contribution underscores and elaborates a "bi-polar conception of the transference." At one pole are the patient's expectations that the transference will be a repetition of the original experiences of selfobject failure, while at the other pole are the patient's need for the analyst to serve as a source of healthy and growth-promoting selfobject responsiveness.

The second chapter in this section, by Morton and Estelle Schane, begins by noting that Kohut himself always argued for an integration of ego psychology and self psychology. Later they suggest that the personality as a whole should be seen from the viewpoint of the model of the bipolar self, of which the tripartite model is a subsector.

The first formal discussion is by Jule Miller. Although appreciative of the efforts by Stolorow and the Schanes, he feels they have not sufficiently acknowledged the extensive efforts of Kohut himself in integrating his ideas with those of classical psychoanalysis. He shares with us Kohut's remarks in response to a clinical vignette he presented to Kohut. This vignette well illustrates Kohut's approach to "classical" (drive-defense) clinical material, seeing it in the context of an "intermediate sequence" resulting from a rupture in the selfobject unit.

The second formal discussion is by Robert Leider. Leider also has much praise for these two papers, but ultimately he cannot agree with their central theses. In response to Stolorow's paper, he questions the utility of the concept "intersubjective field," a concept that is at the core of Stolorow's recent work. Although Leider agrees with much of Stolorow's critique of psychoanalysis, he feels that the introduction of a concept of the intersubjective field is already contained in Kohut's concept of complementarity with a hierarchical clinically based model. In regard to the Schanes' paper, Leider makes the distinction between clinical phenomena and clinical concepts and goes on to disagree with the Schanes' proposal that the way to theoretical integration is to expand the concept of the bipolar self and find a place within some sector of it for a "sanitized" version of the tripartite model. Leider concludes that the tripartite model no longer can be sustained because its central concept of motivation is the "drive."

The next section, on development, spotlights a contribution by Barbara Fajardo. She discusses constitutional factors in the formation of self in early life by reporting the results of her research with premature infants. Among the many important points of her paper, she counters the environmentalist bias of self-psychological theory. She states, "It does not seem that the differences among our developing children can be sufficiently accounted for by variations in the empathic capaci ties of their mothers."

Michael Basch bases his discussion of Fajardo's paper on the cru cial metapsychological concept of the brain as an information-processing organ in which the effective ordering of experience (input) is the centrally relevant issue. From this vantage point he is able to refine, and at the same time distinguish, the metapsychological com prehension of empathy, on one hand, and selfobject experience, on the other. Basch also deduces from metapsychological criteria that the "self-system" encompasses human behavior at all stages of life, "whether prenatal or postnatal." In this context he adds that he re jects Stern's concept of the "emergent self" because he believes that the self and its functions are already in evidence in the first two months of life.

Estelle Schane, in her discussion of Fajardo's paper, takes a differ ent tack from Basch by relying on Stern's concepts of early infancy and in particular the emergent self to discuss the role of selfobject rela tionships in early life.

Section Four begins with David Terman's "Optimim Frustration: Structuralization and the Therapeutic Process." It is a lengthy contri bution that includes a section on developmentalists' views of change and a section detailing therapeutic change in a clinical setting. His major thesis is that Kohut's theory of "structure building" as resulting from "optimal frustration" is in fundamental error. He ends his paper by stating, "I suspect that internalization and structure formation have little to do with frustration." He agrees with Bacal's concept of "op timal responsiveness" and its emphasis on the appropriate ways an analyst may respond in accordance with the patient's phase-appro priate, individually specific requirements for growth or repair. He also agrees with Bacal that "we cannot assume that all internalizing process es occur through frustration."

Bacal, in his discussion of Terman's paper, begins by affirming his agreement with the major points. Bacal and Terman both reject the concept of optimal frustration as leading to structure building ("cure"). It seems to me to try to track down what is *the* curative element in psychotherapy or psychoanalysis is like trying to determine what is *the* central factor in a plant's growth: Is it the sunlight, or the rain, or perhaps the soil in which the plant is anchored? To single out one of these as more important than the others is, of course, absurd. Many factors contribute to a plant's growth, just as many factors contribute to the curative process in psychotherapy or psychoanalysis. However, we must not reject Kohut's ideas of structure formation too quickly. A major problem that has been insufficiently appreciated, I believe, is that the concept of "structure" is a rank metaphor. It is a metaphor taken from building construction, in which a shaky top floor ("mature self") is unstable and needs the building's foundation strengthened. There is now little doubt that the concept of "optimal responsiveness," rather than the ego-psychological "abstinence," is what is necessary for the mobilization of the unfolding of the archaic transferences. My own belief is that the concept of optimal frustration, that is, the disruption and reinstitution of the archaic self-selfobject transference bonds, contributes to a cure by slowly altering the "patterns of expectation" or "expectational sets." The metaphor "structure building" needs to be relocated into the metapsychological domain of information-processing models of the brain.

Bernard Brandchaft's "A Case of Intractable Depression" is the next major contribution. This lengthy description of a clinical psychoanalysis is a welcome addition to the self-psychological literature. Although there is a plethoria of clinical vignettes illustrating this point or that throughout the literature, lengthy case studies are few and far between. Not only is Brandchaft's case a clinical gem with important theoretical implications, but also that it is accompanied by three sophisticated discussions underscores the benefit of its publication in a volume such as this. Each of the discussants, Anna Ornstein, Paul Tolpin, and Ernest Wolf, adds to and deepens Brandchaft's magnificent clinical study.

The final section takes up self-psychological contributions in the applied psychoanalytic domain. The annual conferences have deemphasized self-psychological contributions in the applied area; none of the three essays in this section was presented at the San Diego conference. The first essay is Howard and Margaret Baker's self-psychological exploration of Arthur Miller's *Death of a Saleman*. Their essay is excellent in both its theoretical sophistication and exhaustive attention to detail. The next essay is Carl Rotenberg's "Selfobject Theory and the Artistic Process." It is an in-depth study based on the application of the concept of the self-selfobject unit to the visual arts. His emphasis is on explicating the formal properties rather that the narrative content of the works. His contribution should be seen as affirming Kohut's notions of "cultural selfobjects" mediated at the symbolic level, and illustrating that selfobjects are not always functions fulfilled by the presence of other humans. Marion Solomon's "Treatment of Narcissistic Vulnerability in Marital Therapy" is the final essay. Her work is an important attempt to expand clinical self-psychological theory beyond the individual psychotherapeutic situation. Such areas as couples therapy and marital counseling cry out for a self-psychological treatment framework.

What is clearly conveyed by this volume is the scholarly excellence and high level of contribution that self psychology continues to make to clinical and applied psychoanalysis. What cannot be fully conveyed is the excitement of the conferences themselves. More than once I've reflected that this must have been what it was like in physics for the first two decades of the 20th century: a whole new way of seeing the world has been offered, and a whole new era has begun.

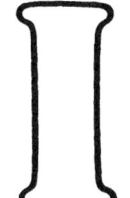

Supervision
with Kohut

Chapter 1

Heinz Kohut as Teacher and Supervisor: A View from the Second Generation

Robert M. Galatzer-Levy

The problem was not that he was a patient—it was that he was just too short. Yet the little man in a bathrobe, standing, waiting in front of the nursing station in corridor A-3 of Billings Hospital had Heinz Kohut's face, a face I knew well from the dust jacket of *The Analysis of the Self*. It seemed impossible that this diminutive person could be the master psychoanalyst, the author of brilliant insights, whose theoretical fluency and compassionate understanding pervaded the book I was carefully studying.

Revolutions in science, large and small, occur not in the pages of research journals, nor on the platforms of scientific conferences. They pervade the lives of scientists, affecting everything from our most abstract thoughts to our self-regard and feelings toward others. The psychology of scientists at the forefront of scientific revolutions has been dramatically described. Most scientists, however, engage in "normal science," the elaboration and exploration of the paradigms whose initial formulation constitutes a scientific revolution.

Like psychological normalcy, the relatively smoothly functioning processes of "normal" scientific work call themselves to our attention less urgently than the atypical events of revolution. The working scientist has integrated so much into his pursuit, so inconspicuously, that

My thanks to Michael Basch, Bertram Cohler, Hannah Decker, Susan Heineman, Jerome Kavka, George Klumpner, Eva Sandberg, Alice and Morris Sklansky, Charles Strozier, and Paul Tolpin for their comments on previous drafts of this paper.

the richness of the activity is easily missed. Even so, mementos of the psychological sources of the scientist's work can be found everywhere—portraits of the teachers who embody his ideals, crumbling bindings of canonical texts, in his love and hatred of colleagues, in a style of discourse that leaps the boundaries of his discipline and is used to explain everyday occurrences.

Kohut (1976) observed that psychoanalytic groups provide exceptional opportunities to study group processes. I began systematically studying psychoanalysis just as Kohut's ideas were coming to prominence. In this paper, by recalling the experience of a beginning analyst in that period, I mean to enlarge our understanding of how new ideas affect the analytic community. I mean neither to evaluate Kohut's ideas nor to examine criticisms and extensions of his work, but rather to study group processes as manifest in one member of a group, myself.

THE REVOLUTION

A revolution in psychoanalysis began in Chicago in the sixties. It was part of a growing dissatisfaction with classical analysis in both its theoretical and its clinical aspects. Though the ultimate effects of this movement are still unknown, its revolutionary character is clear. Most of the phenomena Kuhn (1964) has associated with paradigm[1] shift can be observed in the emergence of self psychology.

Like all new paradigms, self psychology has done more than explain things that are inexplicable or only awkwardly encompassed in older theories. It has also shifted attention away from phenomena for which it is ill suited. The informal, day-to-day thinking of people involved in this new psychology differs from those using the older modes of thought. Whereas the lunchtime conversation and hallway observations of a "classical" analyst include pleased references to some hidden erotic meaning, those using the self psychology paradigm note, with equal glee, the everyday evidence of attempts to keep the self intact and alive.

All analysts are able to formulate clinical phenomena in terms of the psychology of drives, but self psychologists are most likely to be satisfied by explanations in terms of the newer paradigm. They regard drive psychology explanations in the same way that post-Copernican astronomers viewed epicentric computations of the planet's positions—historically interesting, sometimes practical, but fundamentally unsatisfactory.

---

[1] I am using the term paradigm to refer to a framework in which one looks at ideas and information. As I use it, it has no connotations of rigidity or absoluteness, and a level of abstractness is not implied by the term.

There has been a shift in canonical texts. For those deeply influenced by Kohut, his written and verbal statements have largely replaced those of Freud.[2] Beyond its intellectual value, the concern with what Kohut actually did and thought represents an attempt to clarify his embodiment of the self psychology ideal. It parallels the minor industry of Freud biographies, which is a continuation of the culturally universal activity of describing the lives of saints, heroes, and villains.

There is now a group of analysts with a shared self psychology vocabulary, who frequently cite one anothers' work, collaborate in administrative activities, have formed personal bonds, and regard themselves as a community. For better or worse, the psychology of the self is revolutionary in psychoanalysis; it established a new disciplinary matrix and scientific community within psychoanalysis. Its development meets most of the criteria set forth by Kuhn for a scientific revolution.

Having argued for self psychology's revolutionary status, I now want to look at its quieter development as a normal science. The experience of the first generation after a scientific revolution is perhaps particularly illuminating because the processes by which the new paradigm becomes stabilized and transformed into a normal status can be observed. I belong to such a generation.

Anyone writing about his own experiences is faced with many dilemmas. I want to tell enough about my own experience to clarify the psychology of my position. At the same time, I wish to protect my privacy for personal and professional reasons. Little will be said therefore about my experience as an analysand—an unfortunate omission because, clearly, an analyst's ideas are profoundly influenced by his own experiences on the couch. The informal remarks of colleagues and friends are essential to a full history but were never intended for publication and might embarrass them in print. Where necessary, I have used such remarks in disguise and without attribution. Likewise, case material has been disguised. These compromises will doubtless leave both the serious student of psychoanalytic history and the simply curious dissatisfied. Obviously, anonymity and disguise are impossible when discussing Kohut himself. Some of what I have to say about him will doubtless affront certain readers. My goal is to describe a situation as I understand it. It would be an assault on Kohut's memory to present an unrealistic, simplified or bowdlerized picture of him.

---

[2]A transitional phase in this process can be seen in the efforts of some self psychologists, most notably Kohut himself, to refer to Freud's writings and demonstrate the continuity of self psychology with Freud's work.

FIRST ENCOUNTERS

When I spied Heinz Kohut, patient, in the corridors of Billings Hospital, I was a first-year psychiatric resident. I entered the psychiatric residency program at the University of Chicago in the summer of 1971, fresh from medical school. Although I knew I wanted to be an analyst, I still wished to please my very biologically oriented (and therefore antianalytic) teachers at Washington University. So I chose a department with a supposedly eclectic approach. Daniel Freedman, the new chairman, despite periodic avowals of interest in psychoanalysis, was so consistently antagonistic to analysts, analytic training, and analytic ideas that what had been a fine analytic department was gradually losing much of its distinguished analytic faculty. "Standard" analytic concepts and techniques were the particular nemesis of Freedman. The full-time analysts in the department, with the exception of Harry Trosman, were all profoundly influenced by thinking outside the mainstream of contemporary psychoanalysis. Several of them were particularly influenced by the work of Harry Stack Sullivan. Much time was devoted to attacking "downtown" analysts who, after a period of worship at the temple of Freud and Hartmann, greedily practiced a rigid and intellectually unsound version of psychoanalysis. Nonetheless, most of the teaching was done by analysts and candidates. In this atmosphere, ideas that were perceived as contrary to "orthodox" analysis were particularly welcome.

As my first experience as a psychiatric resident in the summer of 1971, I found myself studying emergency room psychiatry with Leonard Elkun, who was then a candidate at the Chicago Institute. Emergency psychiatry was a limited affair—making referrals, occasionally hospitalizing patients, and prescribing neuroleptics. The patients, however, demonstrated all kinds of pathology and provided vivid illustrations of analytic concepts. Elkun, in his enthusiasm for analysis, had us read Schafer's (1964) *Aspects of Internalization* and Kohut's (1971) *Analysis of the Self*. Morning rounds were a heady mixture of management questions, applications of the concept of "primary-process presences" and "selfobjects" to clinical vignettes, and metapsychological debates. I was delighted.

It must be admitted that this delight had little to do with the scientific merit or psychiatric value of the material. After four years of medical school, where a sophisticated chain of reasoning had two steps, it was wonderful to return to the complex arguments that had pleased me so much as an undergraduate and graduate student. In addition, since my previous psychiatric reading had been limited to a few books by Freud and various articles on descriptive psychiatry, I credited Kohut and Schafer with all the developments of modern analytic theory. Kohut's Germanic prose, with its parenthetical remarks and asides to potential critics, seemed reminiscent of the rigorous mathematical discourse I had left behind to study medicine.

Like many analytically untrained readers of Kohut, I consistently mistook the rapidly forming and transient selfobject relations seen in brief patient encounters for the elaborated selfobject transferences observed in analyses.[3] This had a great advantage. What could have been fatiguing administrative situations became exciting adventures on the frontiers of depth psychology.

It was in the midst of this experience that I sighted Heinz Kohut in the halls of Billings Hospital. As I came to appreciate later, the University of Chicago, and particularly the medical center, were a kind of home for Kohut. He had literally lived there as a resident. It was there that he received his neurological and psychiatric training, and there that he continued to teach throughout his life. His actual home was located in the Cloisters, an apartment building adjacent to the university campus and occupied by some of the university's most distinguished faculty. It was at the university's Billings Hospital that he sought medical care for himself and there that he died.

Though I did not see Kohut for another year, his presence was constant. The seminars held at his home, for senior residents, were generally regarded as the best teaching experiences in the program and were widely discussed among us. Moreover, working with very ill patients in the emergency room and inpatient services, I encountered fragmentation and restitution of the self and evidence of failed selfobjects every day. A particularly telling experience for me was co-leading a therapeutic group for acute schizophrenics and their families at the Illinois State Psychiatric Institute, where the university operated a research ward. There I saw, in blatant form, how the most elementary

---

[3]The confusion of these rapidly forming (and dissolving) selfobject relations with the selfobject transferences observed in analyses seems to me to be one of the major sources of difficulty in the appreciation of Kohut's work within the analytic community. It is also a source of its overvaluation by dynamically oriented students and nonanalysts. Many of the phenomena of selfobject relatedness can be observed in ordinary interpersonal interactions and brief psychotherapies. Beginning students often believe that these phenomena represent the depth of the personality. They are delighted to find a system that explains their clinical findings in the very roots of personality formation. In some analytically oriented clinics, the diagnosis of narcissistic personality disorder was for a long time applied to virtually any nonpsychotic patient. The analyst, on the other hand, accustomed to the idea that what is profound must be deeply hidden—and not having recently reread the "Purloined Letter"—tends to reject Kohut's findings precisely because these phenomena are so readily observable. They are then treated as "mere" defense and resistance.

sorts of selfobject functioning repeatedly broke down, leading to the rapid emergence of fragmentation and primitive emergency restitutions in response.

These experiences aroused my interest in self psychology, but they also led me to question Kohut's sharp distinctions between narcissistic personality disorders, borderline states, and psychoses. Sullivan's (1962) remark that "schizophrenics are more human than otherwise"— the observation that much of the time schizophrenics have relatively coherent experiences and that psychotic symptoms, though more striking to the observer, are not the core of these patients' personalities— was more in tune with what I saw than Kohut's idea of a personality fundamentally destroyed. Years later it was this belief that led me, with Kohut's supervisory help and support, to undertake the analysis of manic-depressive patients.

When I became a second-year resident, Kohut's ideas took on new significance for me. My first assignment was to the university's Student Mental Health Service. Kohut's thinking pervaded the service's offices in a converted Hyde Park six-flat. The patients, seen in minuscule offices tucked away in permanently "temporary" arrangements, seemed engaged in a perpetual litany about failed selfobjects and the threats of depletion and fragmentation. Moreover, Betty Kohut worked at the service as a psychiatric social worker. Her personal warmth and charm seemed to me to be empathy incarnate. At conferences she remarked on specific aspects of cases and avoided broad theoretical formulations. In this she contrasted sharply with her husband, who moved rapidly from specific case material to broad generalizations about types of patients, human development, and therapeutic principles. Since many of the case discussions centered on Kohut's ideas, she had endless opportunities to hear often quite undigested and incorrect impressions of her husband's work from residents, consultants, and social workers. She maintained an admirable restraint, generally not correcting the many odd attributions to her husband. I remember only one instance—after someone had proposed a harshly confrontational intervention, supposedly based on Kohut's work, she gently said that she doubted that Heinz had meant what the resident understood.

Like the work with inpatients, psychotherapy with college and graduate students provided many chances to observe the vicissitudes of narcissism. Here again, however, the difference between superficially disturbed narcissistic balance and situations where the personality is dominated by disorders of narcissistic depletion and threatened fragmentation escaped me and most of my colleagues. The patients who came to Student Mental Health were mostly successful young people who were blocked in some developmental task or who had suffered a recent psychological insult, such as the end of a relationship or poor academic performance. As with all people seeking help, their self-esteem was lowered. Often, addressing that loss of self-esteem very early in the therapy was useful. Indeed, the brief therapies of these students tended to follow a standard scenario—a very distressed young person, with seemingly major pathology, rapidly pulled himself together in response to minimal empathic understanding by the therapist. These patients seemed to form relationships with elements of narcissistic transferences to their therapists—feeling sustained in a good feeling about themselves by the therapist's interest and appreciation of them or admiring the therapist and believing they could themselves be vital because of their relationship to him. As I later came to appreciate, however, these selfobject transferences differed from those observed in disorders of the self. The resistance to entering into these transferences and even to avowing them was minimal. The characteristic countertransference difficulties (Kohut, 1971) stimulated by being used as a selfobject were absent. In fact, most therapists greatly enjoyed their work at Student Mental Health. The patients were quite insensitive to the therapists' empathic failures and only minimally affected by separations. These often quite healthy people were skilled in temporarily using the therapists to support them as they accomplished developmental tasks. The relationship to the therapist was like other relationships of late adolescence, intense but relatively brief.[4]

While working at Student Mental Health, I saw the first of a group of patients who were to interest me and for whom I found the insights of self psychology useful. A graduate student whose life had for years been an endless round of "workups" for the rare, hard-to-diagnose,

---

[4]Offenkrantz and Tobin (1975) assert that such therapies work by artificially raising self-esteem. In turn, they say, this results in improved daily functioning and continued rise in self-esteem from the forthcoming approbation. The result is the establishment of a new and better narcissistic equilibrium. This explanation seems unsatisfactory. Instead, I think we see in this type of therapy a variant of the typical selfobject relations of late adolescence. People are temporarily used to provide support for various developmental tasks. In such relationships, the selfobject is not needed for the overall good functioning of the individual, as in disorders of the self. Rather, it supports temporarily enfeebled aspects of the personality, particularly those which are developing.

Although Kohut often spoke of the independent line of narcissistic development, analytic explorations have focused almost exclusively on the pathology of the first years of life. Kohut's (1971) eloquent statements about mature narcissism do not appear to have been generated from analytic material. The details of the line of narcissism and selfobject functioning following the first years of life, particularly during adulthood, have not been adequately described. Such a description is one of the important jobs for self psychology.

and fatal illness, periarteritis nodosa, came to the service. I chose to comment only on the student's experience: to verbalize, as best I could, how he felt. I avoided the idea that his concerns were unrealistic—in a psychological sense, they were not. Nor did I interpret his symptoms as having a hidden meaning. Sticking to this position for only two or three sessions resulted in a startling remission of symptoms. Other aspects of my patient's development, which had been arrested for at least ten years, took major strides.

Over the next several years, I saw 14 other patients with moderate to severe hypochondriacal complaints; 12 of them responded dramatically to similar interventions, with symptom remission or the ability to enter into more intensive therapy. Only the two schizophrenics in this group responded differently. Both became more anxious, and their symptoms worsened (Galatzer-Levy, 1982).

I found the most convincing of the many hypotheses I entertained about these experiences to be that the patients were in a chronic state of threatened fragmentation. They experienced this state as bodily dysfunction. These patients were very ready to enter into selfobject relations that soothed and stabilized them. All that was required was reasonably accurate empathy with their situations, without pejorative confrontations about the metaphor they used to think about themselves. I came to view initial negative responses and difficulties in emotionally understanding my patients as primarily difficulties in myself rather than the patients' pathology.

My work with this form of treatment is an instance of normal science proceeding in the matrix of a new working paradigm, self psychology. Although the work itself was not theoretically novel, it was not, at the time, simply an application of Kohut's ideas to a particular group of patients. With the subsequent elaboration of self psychology, a good resident might be expected to come up with these ideas with a little guidance. Today the situation is like that in other sciences, in which the early research problems of the field become chapter-end exercises well within the abilities of students because the paradigm has been more adequately worked out.

When I wrote about my experiences with hypochondriacs, I used Kohut's ideas extensively, but I did not take them as gospel. Rather, my findings seemed to fit naturally into a self psychology paradigm. I struggled with Kohut's ideas and competing formulations. I tried to provide enough data to support my clinical generalizations, even if I could not find a theory that explained my findings. The self psychology paradigm, at the point I was using it to examine my data, included a description of the dynamics of hypochondriasis, a description of selfobject transferences, and an ideal of empathic immersion as the principal mode of understanding. A clear conceptualization of defense and restitution was not yet part of the paradigm and would have made my work much easier.

What was most important, and perhaps most subtle, was Kohut's influence on my clinical attitude. A critical aspect of my clinical work with hypochondriacs was not confronting them with the nonorganic nature of their concerns. Though I did not realize it then, I and many of my colleagues were influenced by Kohut's expanded vision of analytic neutrality. Analysts have always been ambivalent about neutrality. By examining patients' minds with objectivity, it is possible for both analyst and patient to become aware of ever larger areas of the personality. Any judgmental attitude on the analyst's part interferes with this examination. But isn't the work of analysis to cure the patient by bringing repressed infantile ideas to consciousness, where they are brought into contact with mature, realistic thinking and so corrected? Hardly a neutral position. Furthermore, certain ideas, such as deviant perceptions of external reality, seem so dangerous that the analyst feels impelled to confront the patient with their unrealistic nature, even if this disrupts the analytic process. Kohut thought differently about these matters.

Kohut consistently taught that confronting patients with "reality" interferes with the psychotherapist's empathic position. As a resident, I presented a case of a talented and severely disturbed young musician who finally got a job in his field. One day his employer demanded that he compose a piece of "elevator music." He came to his hour enraged and adamant about quitting the job immediately. Because he was broke and jobs in music are hard to find, I was tempted to try to persuade him to stick with it and bring his grandiosity into better compliance with "reality." Instead, I told him that I understood that work under these circumstances was intolerable. He became calmer, although later that evening he resigned the job. The outcome is worth noting because it is typical of such situations. Although the patient resigned an apparently desirable job, he immediately found work which was more rewarding, both practically and psychologically.[5]

---

[5]It is humbling and increases one's appreciation of psychological reality to observe how often patients' "unrealistic" behavior has positive external results when the decisions come from a self in narcissistic equilibrium. Retrospectively, it often emerges that patients knew more than they said, so these outcomes are not so mysterious. In this case, the patient actually had considerable information about the other job at the time of our session. The therapist's idea that he knows more about reality is often not only antithetical to an analytic position and indicative of hubris, but simply wrong.

Kohut approved of my intervention. He believed that attempts to "educate" the patient about practical realities, no matter how tactful, result in empathic breaks, which almost always cause more damage than what the patient does. Recurrently, Kohut disapproved of tactics designed to "correct" the patient's ideas about internal or external reality.[6]

THE SEMINAR

My first sustained exposure to Kohut himself was in his case seminar for advanced residents at the University of Chicago. I attended this seminar from the summer of 1972 through the spring of 1974. The seminar met in the evening, on the first Wednesday of each month, in the study of Kohut's apartment in the Cloisters. The residents joked that it was our Wednesday evening circle, referring to the early meetings of psychoanalysts in Freud's waiting room. Years later, it was an education in subjective reality to read a *New York Times* reporter's description of the surrounding neighborhood. Where she saw the teeming streets of Chicago's South Side, I perceived a campus epitomizing academia. The Cloisters is located opposite the University Laboratory School's playing field, in an area that attracted not only university faculty, but many psychoanalysts, including George Pollock, the Chicago Institute's president, Therese Benedek, and Charles Kligerman. The building itself, with its central courtyard, large, gracious apartments, and tiny, slow-moving elevators, has an old-fashioned, European

---

[6]It is important to note that Kohut did not mean that the therapist should overlook his own needs and wishes in response to the patient's need to see reality in his own terms. Kohut charged high fees and took long vacations. Although he thought a patient's delay in paying fees should be tolerated and understood as a communication through action rather than confronted or viewed as evidence of superego lacunae, he advocated not insisting on prompt payment *only* if the therapist could conveniently afford the delay. Similarly, he described his distaste for working with a patient who repeatedly called in the middle of the night threatening suicide. It is not the therapist's job, in Kohut's view, to put up with extremely unpleasant behavior. It is, however, his job to recognize that he is likely to fail his patient psychologically in the process. The idea is not to blame the patient for the need but to interpret the failure rather than attempt to end the demand through reference to some supposed normative standard. The notion that it is the therapist's duty to directly meet the psychological needs of patients has led to antitherapeutic enactments by some of Kohut's followers and unjust criticism by some of his detractors, but it was not part of Kohut's teaching.

Indeed, Kohut's position contrasts sharply with Winnicott's way of working with patients with early developmental pathology, with whom he frequently enacted the demanded "holding" and caretaking (Little, 1985).

charm. I had a sense of visiting another era when I went to Kohut's apartment.

Dominated by a large etching of Freud looking wise and somewhat disapproving, Kohut's study was a small room, overcrowded when ten or so residents attended the seminar. The Freud icon literally hung over us as we presented cases. A copy of the *Standard Edition* and the volumes of *The Psychoanalytic Study of the Child* occupied a small bookshelf, while books like *Modern English Usage* and *The Chicago Manual of Style* were on a shelf above a writing desk. I assumed that Kohut wrote there and was amazed that such important work could be done in such ordinary surroundings.

Kohut, although invariably courteous, was slightly fastidious about getting mud on the carpets and hanging coats neatly. I am still unclear about what was his obsessionalism and what was my awe. He wanted us to be comfortable, but he was not facile in promoting this.

During each session, residents presented cases in treatment or diagnostic consultations. Kohut listened for a while and then discussed the case from a self psychology viewpoint. To those of us who had "caught on" to self psychology, the content of these discussions was unsurprising. This predictability was exacerbated by the residents' tendency to choose material that lent itself to self psychology explanations. (Kohut often expressed skepticism about his clinical impression of the incidence of self disorders, since he knew patients and supervisees sought him out because of his interest in these conditions.)

If residents referred to classical theory in their presentations, Kohut acknowledged this and began by describing how the case material could be understood in terms of drives and defenses. These explanations consistently lacked power. There was no question that Kohut believed these explanations represented good psychodynamic formulation, but they usually had the character of strawmen.[7] By this I do not mean that he omitted some potentially useful theoretical viewpoint. Rather, the sort of interpretation that makes the listener think,

---

[7]It seems most improbable to me that Kohut could have achieved his high status as a "classical" analyst with formulations like those he presented to the residents. Perhaps the combined needs for condensation, his lack of enthusiasm for the older ideas, and a wish to show self psychology in the best light resulted in these uninspired renditions of classical concepts. Certainly the reports that Kohut was a brilliant teacher of classical ideas are inconsistent with what I later observed. Is it possible that Kohut was all along working within the context of the rather weak version of classical analysis that he presented? If so, how could he ever have been enthusiastic about it? It might then be less surprising that he abandoned it. Here, it would be very valuable for colleagues who knew Kohut well before he developed self psychology to describe their experiences with him.

"That's right! I never thought of that!" was missing. Kohut asserted that they were unsatisfactory and went on to explanations and recommendations in terms of self psychology. He never recommended interpretation of motives or defenses that were out of the patient's awareness. Instead, he focused on the therapist's increasing empathy for his patient's position.

Kohut was an extraordinarily convincing speaker. His voice was resonant, and he spoke fluently in long, complex sentences. He was often theatrical, and his timing was magnificent. Affects were evoked through intonation, not concrete imagery. The tone of voice most often evoked the analyst's benign and supportive attitude. It was easy to imagine the effects of his manner on a patient.

For many of us, Kohut's speech contributed to his charisma. To this day, reading Kohut, I imagine his voice and intonation, which change his complex, abstract prose into something emotionally evocative and nearly poetic. It was startling to realize that despite the charm and conviction with which he delivered his remarks, Kohut's statements sometimes did not stand close scrutiny. Once, for instance, he discussed the confirmation of a reconstruction about a patient's early development through the patient's observation of his "now ancient parents." It sounded great, but on leaving the seminar it occurred to me that these "ancients" were probably people in their forties.

Reconstructions are a weak point in self psychology. Too often they seem to blame parents for the child's pathology and to ignore the child's activity in forming both the perceived and actual behavior of the parent. I am well aware that Kohut was talking about the patient's *experience* of the parent. Nonetheless, the question of why the patient experienced the parent in the way he did was never explored. The implicit answer thus became that the patient experienced the parent that way because that was the way the parent was.

In the seminar, Kohut consistently reconstructed the developmental consequences of parental pathology and unavailability. The data for such reconstructions were the patient's conscious views of his current life and recollections from latency and adolescence. Kohut freely described parental responses on the basis of such evidence. It could be argued that Kohut was only doing what analysts often do—generalizing from psychoanalytic reconstructions carefully worked out, through the analysis of transference, to data arising from other situations. It might also be said that he was attending to the patient's subjective experience and exclusively reconstructing such experience. It might even be said that he was modeling empathic understanding of patients. Yet, in retrospect, I am left with the uneasy feeling that he was quite certain about these reconstructions and wanted us to share his conviction.

Generally, even when he disagreed with a resident, Kohut was kindly and tactful in his discussion. But he was in no sense egalitarian. He believed in the correctness of his views, and his manner with us was that of patient mentor rather than a fellow explorer.

I saw him get angry only once during the seminar. A resident, clearly wanting to show up analytic types, presented a neurological case. He had the ill-concealed motive of demonstrating how ignorant analysts were of neurology. He described a young woman with multiple sclerosis and psychiatric symptoms and asked Kohut to provide a differential diagnosis between the organic components of these symptoms, the effects of medication, and psychogenic factors. "After all," he said, "this is a general psychiatric case conference."

Kohut smiled, not at all nicely, and observed that it had been thirty years since he had resigned from his assistant professorship in neurology to study psychiatry, so his recollections on this matter were not "entirely fresh." He proceeded to discuss the differential diagnosis beautifully, in the manner of a sophisticated attending neurologist, periodically glaring at the red-faced resident. (The only other time I saw Kohut manifestly angry was after he read a review of *The Restoration of the Self*. He said he did not really mind if it took time for his ideas to be understood, but "willful stupidity" did not deserve publication.)

Kohut was an extraordinarily clear and interesting teacher, so his ideas were widely discussed among the residents. The sense of being at the fountainhead of emerging ideas, which the residents shared with Kohut, gave Kohut's teaching a unique vitality. At the same time, as I have already suggested, his authoritative voice could lend credence to ideas that were simply wrong, particularly when they were emotionally appealing. It was not uncommon to leave a Kohut seminar having heard a lovely analogy, only to realize that, while the analogy was convincing, it was factually mistaken. An example from his written work will give the flavor of this phenomenon. In *How Does Analysis Cure?* Kohut compares the expert self psychologist analyst to the "master pianist who will for a moment think of finger positions and the like. . . . Like the pianist who devotes all his attention to the conception of the work he performs and to the artistic message it transmits, so also the experienced self psychologist." The type of psychological phenomenon Kohut wishes to describe is clear, and the image of the virtuoso pianist appealing. Unfortunately, it is simply wrong. The concert pianist spends enormous amounts of time working over, perfecting, and reworking his technical skills. During a performance he does not think in words either about technical or artistic matters but rather "hears and then plays the music" (Schnabel, 1942; Mach, 1980).[8]

The capacity to evoke belief, even among sophisticated and skeptical listeners, was an important aspect of Kohut's personality. Was Kohut, then, a charismatic personality? Certainly, like many outstanding teachers, he inspired idealization. We tended to accept ideas simply because they were his. The grandiosity that is an aspect of the charismatic individual was clearly present in Kohut, though in modified and subtle form.

Kindness and courtesy were important aspects of Kohut's personality. When I sent out notices as I began private practice, only two people wrote back wishing me well. Kohut's brief encouraging note was most welcome to a young man beginning what seemed an uncertain and difficult course.

Stolorow and Atwood (1979) demonstrate that psychological theories grow out of the needs of their inventors. It would be easy to speculate on Kohut's personal motives for developing the psychology of the self, but to do so meaningfully would require a greater knowledge of Kohut than I have. It is nonetheless interesting to wonder whether his observation of selfobject transferences reflected some aspect of his character. Transference, as I now understand it, is the product of the psychological needs of the patient and the actuality of the analyst (often

---

[8]It is no accident that this same passage caught the attention of Wallerstein (1985) as an example of Kohut's "condescending tone" or—described from another viewpoint—Kohut's insufficiently regulated grandiosity. Clinically we know that failures in reality testing are associated with such grandiosity, and I think this is an example of a subtle failure of this kind. It is typical of such failures that they leave the audience (which wants to believe anyway) at least temporarily convinced of their validity.

Several readers, who otherwise were very much in sympathy with the material presented here, believe it is I, not Kohut, who is mistaken about how musical virtuosos operate, despite the many written and oral statements in support of my view by professional musicians. Assuming I am correct, what is the source of Kohut's error and the resistance to my observation? First, there is of course the pleasure of the grand image of the virtuoso, untroubled by the petty details of technique which plague less great men. In addition, Kohut's error may have an idiosyncratic source in that it approximates a position taken by the "romantic" school of musical performance was prevalent in Vienna in the early part of this century. His father may have held such a view or been trained by someone with such a view. Another source of the error is the equation of all work in an area with the moment of fluid performance, when indeed conscious attention to every detail would make performance impossible. I think a romantic view of analytic work may cloud our attention to the many hours of conscious cognitive work reflected in action which seems smooth to us. Finally, we analysts may be confused about how professionals, including ourselves, function optimally. Maybe we should learn from the pianists, who are perpetually perfecting the details of technique.

as affected by the patient). Certainly it is easy to understand how idealization was a common response to his personality in analysis, as it was among his students and colleagues. Mirroring, on the other hand, was not as obvious an aspect of Kohut's personality as I witnessed it. Indeed, one had a sense that while he was able to respond empathically, this did not come particularly easily or naturally to him. Perhaps here Kohut turned a difficulty in his own personality into an asset by examining the effect of that deficit on his patients.

As I have discussed and shared drafts of this paper with more senior colleagues and others who knew Kohut in other contexts, I have heard many tales about a man of considerable insecurity, self-centeredness and "difficulty"; a person quite different from the one I knew. His former students, however, tend to share views similar to mine, in which strong positive feelings and the remains of idealization are modified by the recognition of areas of difficulty, but in which the spirit of personal admiration predominates. In forming a balanced picture of Kohut's personality, both sets of experiences need to be recorded. I think, however, that it is an error to consider the more unpleasant aspects of Kohut's character as somehow more authentic than the admirable aspects of his personality that dominated students' experiences with him. Those aspects were not a false front, but rather a vital aspect of Kohut, which came usefully to the fore in relation to the students whose own development required such an idealizable teacher.[9]

THE CANDIDATE'S VIEW

Increasing fame, interest in spreading his ideas beyond Chicago, illness, and a desire to write all limited Kohut's teaching of analytic candidates by the time I started course work at the Chicago Institute in

---

[9]That Kohut was able to provide for the psychological needs of others in depth is supported by the testimony of one of his patients from days long preceding the development of self psychology. This patient, now a distinguished analyst, recalls that Kohut was an extraordinarily good listener, capable of sustained, intense interest in the details of the patient's life. He also comments that Kohut's interpretations were very close to experience and that a theoretical orientation was not obvious in them.

In discussing a draft of this paper, colleagues have pointed out that both the period of the development of self psychology and the period during which I knew Kohut were also a time when he was chronically and seriously ill. Some analysts noted a marked shift in Kohut's personality with his illness. Others, who knew him well, felt the change was less profound Certainly, Kohut's constant awareness of death influenced the way he presented his ideas and gave urgency to his wish to say what he had to say. In any case, more information about the relationship of Kohut's personality and personal development in relation to his theories would be most welcome.

1975. We listened enviously when more advanced students described the beautiful course in analytic theory that Kohut no longer taught. Even so, Kohut's influence was felt in virtually every class, seminar, and supervision.

For many reasons, I will not detail the effects of Kohut's thinking on my own experience as an analytic patient. Certainly both my analyst and I included self psychology ideas in our thinking, though my analyst was not one of the group closely identified with Kohut. He was, however, able to allow the transference to develop as it might, not interrupting that development with premature interpretations of material as resistance. Were I required to affix theoretical labels to the issues we dealt with, I would say that self psychology issues were worked on extensively in my analysis.

I include this information because in classes it became obvious that candidates' responses to Kohut's work reproduced their own analysts' attitudes toward self psychology. This is a perennial problem in psychoanalysis. Analysts' responses to new ideas are profoundly influenced by unresolved analytic transferences.[10]

Analytic candidates spend years with their classmates. Expectably, feelings grow intense. Our group remained reasonably amicable throughout our training, except in the area of self psychology. Most of the students were in a position similar to my own. Their analysts were not part of the self psychology group, but they were interested in self psychology developments and particularly curious about the clinical applications of self psychology. One candidate was, however, forever sounding the note of danger—that self psychology concepts could be used to resist true analytic insights. After a while, it became almost humorous to listen to his "concern" that "young people like Dr. A. might be seduced by Kohut's ideas." Dr. A., who was perhaps

---

[10]Whether other scientists are better off in this regard is an open question. Transferences to teachers and leaders in the field profoundly influence scientific thinking, and the unanalyzed scientist lacks the opportunity to consciously work through such transferences. On the other hand, the intensity of the scientist's transferences is often considerably less than that of analytic candidates, and transferences are frequently defused among several teachers, so that any one teacher is likely to have a less profound influence in a modern scientific institution than the candidate's analyst. Frequently these transferences are also directed toward idealized leaders of the science. In psychoanalysis, for most analysts, this role is played exclusively by Freud. (A comparable situation existed with Newton for almost 200 years in physics.) Thus a simple comparison of the effects of unresolved transferences on the development of analytic theory to similar phenomena in other sciences is impossible.

One indication that Kohut's own analytic work did adequately address issues of idealization, particularly idealization leading to slavish agreement on ideological issues, is the large number of Kohut's analysands who have developed ideas that disagree with their analysts' in an undefiant fashion.

ten years our senior, is one of the keenest intellects around the Institute, a thoughtful and skeptical individual, who had made research contributions to psychoanalysis. The candidate's attitude was clearly in massive identification with his own analyst.

Like me, many of my classmates had cut their psychiatric teeth on Kohut's work. The result was a peculiar misalignment between certain teachers and candidates. The teachers, thinking they were introducing new and difficult ideas, spent hours gently acquainting us with long-familiar self psychological concepts. The assumption was, even among the self psychologists, that drive theory was baseline analytic thinking and that other ideas, including self psychology, were to be viewed in relation to that theory. What was perhaps a necessary step in the development and pedagogy of self psychology, the careful connection to classical ideas put forward in *The Analysis of the Self*, became a stultifying redundancy in teaching us.

At the same time, though ego and drive psychology were taught in courses in theory, it was rare in the clinical courses to focus sustained attention on decoding symbolism or discovering the drive origins of a psychological phenomenon. One teacher who regularly carried out such a program did it more as an exercise in showing how it could be done than with the conviction that such an approach was clinically useful. I do not recall any of my teachers carrying the conviction that psychology could be understood as a simple playing out of a group of formulas centering on drive development and the vicissitudes of oedipal conflicts. Though Kohut's work was far from universally accepted, a broadened scope of psychoanalytic thinking was employed by the entire faculty, and this clearly was partly the result of the presence of Kohut and his followers within the institute.

We of the second generation had a model in Lou Shapiro, the Institute's former dean and generally recognized master analytic clinician. Shapiro taught a case seminar for second-year candidates. He consistently advocated a position of empathic comprehension as the analytic mode of listening and freely credited Kohut with educating him about the treatment of disorders of the self.

With regard to analytic technique, many of the ideas associated with Kohut's work were common coin among large segments of the faculty. Virtually all the teachers avowed a position that transference should evolve at its own pace, without interruptions and distortions introduced by the analyst's activity. With two exceptions, none of my teachers or supervisors urged the aggressive or intrusive interpretation of defenses and drives. Sam Lipton, who was in no sense a self psychologist, attempted to demonstrate that the rigidly abstinent stand commonly advocated in the literature of the fifties and sixties was neither true to the Freudian tradition nor clinically useful. One of my supervisors, Bernard Kamm, who trained at the Berlin Institute in the thirties and is as classical an analyst as could be imagined, was fond of pointing out that the commonly recommended analyst's silence, so objectionable to many patients, communicated something entirely different in contemporary American culture from what it implied in early 20th-century Europe. Silence to modern Americans, he pointed out, is a sign of disapproval and superiority. In Europe, paternal silence was an approving invitation to speak.

The idea that the analyst should behave with ordinary courtesy and avoid interfering with transference developments by offering premature, pejorative interpretations is logically independent of self psychology theory. It was emphasized by Kohut in *The Analysis of the Self* and reflected his own ideal of analytic method. The idea had thus long been held within our institute; at the same time it gained increased status through Kohut's reassertion. It is interesting to note that willingness to let the transference develop as it may is directly antithetical to Alexander's active technique and thus the equation of the work of these two leaders of the Chicago Institute is particularly ill founded.

Both in class and in supervision, Kohut's ideas aroused the most interest during clinical discussions. Since I was a candidate in both child and adult analysis, by the middle of the third year of training I had six regular supervisors as well as a consultant whom I saw privately. Perhaps because of my own interest in self psychology, I had much opportunity to compare and contrast attitudes held by all these supervisors about self psychology issues.

In the supervisory situation, my teachers expressed much stronger positions for or against self psychology than in the classroom. All strongly urged allowing the material to emerge as it might. Yet each was a strong advocate of one position or another and tended to take the failure of the patient to "spontaneously" develop the "right" transference as an indication of technical errors on my part. At times this became quite distressing. For a time I regularly had two supervisory hours in sequence. One was with an analyst who considered Kohut's ideas antithetical to analytic exploration. He thought that Kohut was advocating a "corrective emotional experience" that led the analyst to play the role of a new and better parent and also to collude in the patient's attribution of his own internal difficulties to the environment. The second supervisor was a close student of Kohut.

However informative in retrospect, at the time it was an awful experience. Within minutes, the first supervisor chastised me for gratifying the patient and interfering with the analysis for what the second supervisor regarded as providing normal empathic understanding. On another day, the second supervisor gently suggested careful self-analysis to discover why I had behaved so unempathically when I followed the technique advocated by my first supervisor. Though each of these supervisors claimed an intellectual openness to other outlooks, when push came to shove, each was convinced of the correctness of his own view. It is inevitable that any serious analyst would take a strong position on Kohut's ideas. It is impossible to work for years with a theoretical orientation, profoundly affecting the lives of our patients, without considerable conviction about the correctness of what we are doing. Yet for a student eager to do well and please his supervisors, and to develop his own conviction about analytic ideas, such diversity in supervisory outlooks creates massive tension. The virtue of having such an experience is that the internal voice of supervisory wisdom is forever accompanied by a healthy skepticism.

The child analytic supervisors were particularly interesting in their responses to Kohut's work. As a group, they were more committed to drive-defense psychology than were my other teachers. They were also far more interested in and influenced by such diverse ideas as observational studies of infants, Kleinian theory, and the work of Margaret Mahler. They were much less likely than analysts who saw only adults to view the child as passively traumatized by the environment and more likely to inquire about the child's active role in the situation. Kohut's emphasis on parental failures did not include this perspective.[11] At the same time, I only once believed the often heard response to Kohut's ideas "but we knew all of that already"—when it came from a child analyst who, though theoretically miles from self psychology, understood very well what the self psychologists were getting at. This is not too surprising. Much of the work of child analysts is with youngsters with serious developmental (borderline) pathology, so as a group we probably have more experience with self pathology than most analysts. In addition, our patients are less compliant and more direct in telling us how we are unuseful.

An important factor in the rejection of self psychology by many child analysts is the disparity between the child's world as observed by the child analyst, both in analysis and in analytically informed child observation, and the child's world described by Kohut. Not unlike Melanie Klein, Kohut described a psychological world of the first year of life that is in many ways sharply at odds with what even the most

---

[11]Kohut's position, which is entirely one of inner subjectivity, is not at all inconsistent with the view that the child actively creates and influences his environment and that, if justice were done, aspects of the child, even his wishes, lead to traumatization. The emotional point of view of the analyst who thinks in this way, however, is radically different and easily discernible in his communication to the patient.

empathic observer sees. When Kohut cited child observations, he was often unconvincing or simply inaccurate. During the residents' seminar, for example, he had occasion to describe the game "This little piggy went to market." In Kohut's version, the toes were wiggled in sequence until, with the words "all the way home," the child was embraced. He interpreted the game as a piece of work on the problem of fragmentation. The attention to the individual toes represented attention to separate body parts and the hug the appreciation of the whole child. Unfortunately, the game is not played in the way Kohut described. Rather, it ends with the adult rapidly moving his hand up the child's leg while tickling him and then tickling the abdomen and sometimes the upper trunk. Usually the child giggles, and often the tickling is continued to the point of stimulating the slightly disorganizing and almost overstimulating laughter characteristic of "ticklish" children.[12] (As with similar factual misstatements by Kohut, I cannot recall anyone ever correcting him. In addition to the question of how Kohut's personality evoked uncritical responses, clearly some source of corrective feedback became unavailable to Kohut.)

In sum, Kohut's presence was felt throughout my training at the Chicago Institute for Psychoanalysis. Questions about the relationship of his work to other theories were a major theme of that training. Powerful, irrational factors, such as unresolved analytic transferences, envy, and the emotional satisfactions of group membership, were obvious determinants of my classmates' and teachers' responses to his work. Sometimes this led to intense creative discourse; at other times it resulted in futile and irrational struggles. For the student trying to find his feet in psychoanalysis, the situation often intensified the anxiety that is often relieved by certitude about theory and ideal technique. But it also provided an atmosphere in which analysis was seen as a creative and developing field—a field to which one might reasonably hope to make a contribution.

KOHUT THE SUPERVISOR

For as long as I can remember, I have wanted to be a scientist. This

---

[12]Admiration and idealization can lead one to doubt the obvious. When I first heard Kohut's description, I wondered if the people I knew, including myself, had somehow gotten involved in a deviant version of this game, one contrary in purpose to what Kohut had in mind. This led me to question many people and watch a lot of little toes being pulled. Every description of the game I heard and all my observations of it were as I described here, quite different phenomenologically from Kohut's and not consistent with his interpretation.

is hardly amazing, since my father, a biochemist, held science as his ideal. As I grew older, the idea of being a scientist evolved from a simple wish to be like my father. When I entered medical and psychiatric training, I assumed I would make intellectual contributions to my field. Starting in medical school, I routinely combined a research interest with almost everything I did professionally. My first papers were descriptive summaries of experiences in the two clinics I helped organize and operate as a medical student, one for an impoverished black community, the other for adolescent drug users (Freiden, Levy, and Harmon, 1970; Levy and Brown, 1971; Levy and Halkas, 1972; Levy, 1973, 1974).

As I began to study psychoanalytic ideas, it was obvious that the theory was in sorry shape. Freud's first sketch of a comprehensive theory of human psychology was treated as completed work, so the outline of his massive project was never filled in. In a sense, working in analytic theory is like being a pioneer in a recently opened wilderness. Even with a moderate knowledge of agricultural techniques, the pioneer has a problem not in finding useful work but in selecting from the riches before him. So, too, the student of analysis with a reasonable knowledge of other fields, whether the sciences or history or literary criticism, is presented with seemingly innumerable possibilities. My training in mathematics and the sciences constantly suggested approaches to the theoretical problems of psychoanalysis, although it has been possible to follow only a small fraction of these ideas to the point of publication.

Contributing significantly to clinical psychoanalysis is much harder. In many areas of clinical work, psychoanalysis is a fairly mature field. Even though problems of verification are perpetually challenging, and new ideas about clinical situations appear frequently, a basically solid group of concepts about clinical matters is shared within the analytic community. Though every patient is unique and every analysis in a sense a research, most of what is found in any analysis has already been described in detail in our literature.

There are also practical difficulties in making clinical contributions. Inevitably personal analytic experience is limited.[13] Many cases, such as those involving colleagues or their families, can be communicated

---

[13] As analyses become longer, analytic patients grow more scarce, and the age of analytic candidates increases, the possibilities for broad personal experience as an analyst decrease. At a recent meeting of analysts who graduated from our institute in the past five years, most had four patients currently in analysis (a figure considerably above the national averages). Assuming an average age of 47 for the group, an average retirement age of 67, and analyses lasting on the average five years, the lifetime analytic experience of my colleagues will involve 20 to 25 analyses. Thus, even in an active analytic community like ours, it is the rare individual who accumulates a truly substantial analytic experience.

only in the most general and circumspect way. Finally, technical innovation and experimentation, as opposed to theoretical invention, entail a responsibility to treat patients to the best of one's abilities. Caution is wise and ethically imperative in applying new and untried methods.[14]

As mentioned earlier, in studying hypochondriacs, I had the experience of trying out a relatively new psychotherapeutic approach described by others. Yet the likelihood of having experiences as an analyst that would contribute substantially to analytic technique, though longed for, seemed slight.

From this perspective, I was more than happy when a young man with manic-depressive illness presented himself for analysis. I have described this case elsewhere (Galatzer-Levy, 1987). In brief, the patient was referred to me after a manic episode. He disliked me and sought treatment elsewhere. Discovering that he disliked the other psychiatrist in the same way he disliked me, he recognized on his own that the dislike must have originated predominantly within himself. He returned to me for treatment. He wanted very much to understand what had happened to him and was dissatisfied, both intellectually and emotionally, with the best biological theories. An analysis was offered with the understanding that it was not a standard technique of treatment and that all I could realistically offer was my serious attempt to understand his psychology.

During his seminar for residents, Kohut had mentioned his own attempt to analyze manic-depressive patients. He said relatively little about this work, except that he had introduced the technical innovation of seeing the patients at the end of the day and allowing the session's length to be determined either by the patient or his own fatigue.[15] He also mentioned that his patients took lithium, but this medication was managed by another physician so as not to confuse the transference.

I telephoned Kohut, told him about my patient, and expressed my wish for his ongoing consultation. He said it sounded very interesting. Kohut mentioned his fee of $100 (at a time when analytic fees

---

[14]It seems preposterous to me to speak of informed consent in this context or, for that matter, any other context involving intense transferences. While it is essential that the analyst not only recommend the treatment he believes best for the patient but also attempt to address the most rational aspect of the patient's character with the difficulties and dangers of undertaking a particular course, it is contrary to everything we know to think that the patient will then make an informed and rational decision based on that information.

[15]This experimental technique, and another instance in which Kohut allowed a terrified patient to grasp his fingers, are the only instances I heard of Kohut's mention deviating from standard analytic procedure in his own work.

ranged from $70 to $80 in Chicago) and said that he understood that the fee was high but that he hoped it caused me no great hardship. I was so pleased to have the chance to work with him that I did not think of objecting.[16]

In the first hour, I told Kohut about the patient's history and our interactions up until that time. The patient had particular difficulty with his family's and the previous psychiatrist's emphasis on the need for him to "adapt to reality." I had responded to his grandiosity and rage at not being appreciated with interpretive indications that I understood the value of his grand ideas and the rage he felt at the oppressive demands that he conform. Not surprisingly, Kohut was thoroughly approving of this approach. As he did regularly in our session, he took brief notes and, after listening to the material, expounded on his ideas about it. Predictably, he understood the material in terms of a self endangered by failures of mirroring. The parents continued into the present the empathic failures that had resulted in the fragile development of my patient's self. Their current behavior was seen as strongly supporting the reconstruction that such failures were recurrent in childhood and infancy.

I was disappointed—Kohut was a Kohutian. I expected new revelations but received only confirmation of my own self psychology formulations. Furthermore, Kohut's formulation failed to address the central problem of the case—why my patient suffered from manic-depressive illness rather than a narcissistic personality disorder. It occurred to me, however, that Kohut could not be blamed for the un satisfactory nature of our first meeting. Given the range of response to his work, he had no way of knowing my familiarity with or respect for self psychology.

I began the next hour by stating that, given his fees, I would ask him what I wanted to know. He laughed warmly. I asked, "Is this crazy? Does it make sense to try to analyze a manic-depressive?" He paused and looked mock-solemn. Then, grinning, he replied, "No, it does not make sense. But then, few things in life worth doing make sense." He went on to say that this was a research analysis, whose therapeutic outcome we could not know in advance or even speculate

---

[16]On reading an earlier draft of this paper, Michael F. Basch observed that this interchange certainly was not about money. Rather, it involved Kohut's demand to be mirrored and my disavowed reluctance to serve as a mirroring selfobject. Kohut's empathy (at least within the metaphor) further complicated the situation. That the interchange remained important to me is evident not only in my decision to report it here, but in the opening of the second session with Kohut. The elaboration of the meaning of such interchanges, which I do not undertake here, may lead to an understanding of both the interpersonal means by which people needing mirroring and people needing to idealize get together, and also the difficulties inherent in such situations.

on with a reasonable degree of certainty. He thought analysis would not harm the patient and certainly nothing else would help him in the way he wanted to be helped, so from the patient's viewpoint it was a reasonable undertaking. More important, it was an opportunity to explore manic-depressive illness analytically. The attempt would contribute to my development as an analyst and to the development of the science of psychoanalysis.[17]

Kohut went on to discuss a personal experience he evidently had had as an advanced candidate. Under the supervision of Max Gitelson, he had attempted to analyze a schizophrenic young man. The analysis had been an utter therapeutic failure, and he thought that the patient was currently chronically hospitalized in a state institution. Nevertheless, Kohut felt he had learned a lot about the patient's psychology in the attempt.

There was something cold in Kohut's description of the sad outcome of this endeavor. His style was more reminiscent of a physical scientist describing a failed, but interesting experiment than of the attitude I am accustomed to from analysts. It was the first time I wondered whether Kohut's interest in empathy did not reflect a relative absence in himself of a spontaneous empathic capacity.[18] Yet, if this

---

[17]Aside from Freud's remarks about his own lack of therapeutic ambition, I have seen little written about two very different sets of conscious motives found among analysts for their work. Some choose analysis because of its therapeutic power, others because of its intellectual satisfactions. These two aspects of analysis are independent—effective therapy can be based in mistaken theory, and accurate understanding need not be therapeutic. Listening closely to my colleagues, I have found not only that most analysts are primarily interested in one or the other of these aspects of analysis, but that they tend to assume that all analysts are motivated in the same way they are. Some amusing failures of understanding arise from such assumptions. Not so amusing is that the idea of a "good analysis" is quite different for these two groups. For the clinically motivated, the therapeutic outcome is most important, so arguments about the validity of methods seem academic and foolish. For the researcher, the intellectual validity of the insights achieved is of great importance, with clinical results being a welcome but not central benefit for the analyst. (Unfortunately, there is yet another group, who might be called the ritualists, whose central concern is no longer with the function of the analysis but rather with the correctness of its form.)

[18]Writing about Kohut's personality in the current atmosphere, in which so much hostility is directed against him and his work, is problematic for someone who admires both the man and his ideas. As with Freud and other analysts, his detractors will doubtless seize on any indications of pathology, especially as related to his work, as a way to attack Kohut and his contributions. One is reluctant to give them ammunition. On the other hand, as Stolorow and Atwood (1979) show, the appreciation of psychoanalytic contributions and their history is enriched by an understanding of the factors in the theorist's personality that contributed to his achievement. Furthermore, it would be clearly contradictory to any understanding we have of creativity to posit that such a major undertaking as the reformulation of psychoanalysis did not come from the depths of Kohut's personality and was not motivated by strong forces within him.

was so, Kohut transformed this deficit into a major scientific advance.

From this point on in the supervision, Kohut and I were very much on the same wavelength. What I needed most from the supervision, and what Kohut consistently provided, was not his specific intellectual understanding of the work, however valuable that was, but his interest and support in psychoanalytic exploration. His capacity to see and value this potential in a young colleague was unique among my teachers.

Kohut was not particularly interested in the details of my novel formulations. For example, as the work progressed, I noticed that my patient both profoundly mistrusted and tended to be unaffected by verbal statements. This observation first led me to the notion that his parents were hypocritical and covered their intense anxieties with neat verbal formulas. Kohut thought this was very much to the point and discussed this idea as evidence for the mother's latent psychosis. Later, however, when I began to understand the same material in terms of a failure in the development of language to communicate about intense affects, Kohut was quite uninterested. He worried that such theoretical interests would interfere with my accurate appreciation of the patient's subjective states.[19]

Kohut was too busy and burdened by his many activities to spend time supporting and acknowledging colleagues on all levels, much less seriously working over new ideas outside his own frame of reference. His writings (like Freud's) paid little heed to his predecessors. He considered his time better spent putting forward his own ideas than recounting their origins. (At times this approach merely led to wounded feelings for those who were not appreciated. At other times, as in his discussion of the historical aspects of guilty and tragic man, Kohut's failure to attend adequately to available scholarly material led to unsound positions, which could easily have been avoided.) Similarly, his limited interest in others' research reflected his preoccupation with advancing his own thoughts.

When I asked him to read a manuscript of mine, he smiled and asked if I knew what a "real Kohutian dream" was. He said he had a recurrent dream in which a man threateningly advanced toward him with one hand behind his back. The classical interpretation clearly had to do with castration, the missing hand, and the danger of retribution. But the Kohutian interpretation was that the man must have a manuscript that he wanted Kohut to read. He then volunteered to read my paper—which, however, I never brought to him.

---

[19]Kohut was consistent in this regard. His dislike of standard formulations of defense operations arose, I think, not because he failed to appreciate that people fool themselves to avoid anxiety, but rather because formulations in these terms inevitably are at odds with subjective experience.

The Use of Interpretation

Kohut's recommendations to me in supervision were uniformly consistent with his published views. The analysis of transference through interpretation was the principal work of analysis. Kohut heartily approved of the following intervention, for example. When, in the session before the first summer vacation, my patient became overtly psychotic, believing that he controlled my mind and exhibiting clear symptoms of mania, I interpreted to him that it was essential to him to control me in this way because my continued interested presence was vital to his existence. No attempt, other than the interpretation, was made to "manage" the situation.

At the same time that transference was central to the analysis, the presence of transference manifestations was not to be sought in Holmesian fashion, according to Kohut. Consistent with his views of the analysis of resistance, any but the most blatant displacements of the transference were not to be interpreted and then only as instances of replacing the failed or lost selfobject. For instance, my patient developed a friendship with a psychiatrist of roughly my age who, like me, was bearded and balding. The friendship revolved around a competitive sport, at which my patient consistently trounced the psychiatrist. An interpretation of displaced competition left both the patient and Kohut cold. Saying, however, that the patient had successfully found someone who filled some of my functions when I was unavailable seemed on track to both (and led to elaborations and new associations from the patient).

Similarly, Kohut believed that dreams should, in this case, be interpreted entirely as representations of self states, that the interpretations should focus on the states of the self represented in the dream, as understood through a universally comprehensible symbolism. The patient's associations were not sought, nor were they given great weight. Kohut emphasized the usefulness of following a series of dreams to monitor the development and stabilization of the self. During the second year of the analysis, my patient had several dreams in anticipation of a break in the analysis. In each he was flying, holding on to the back of the train that brought him to our session. In the first dream he was unable to hold onto the train and fell off into the snow, where he froze. In another he again could not hold on but on letting go was able to continue flying. In the final dreams, he held on to the train with a combination of excitement and terror. Kohut thought that to look for elaborate symbolism or ask for associations in these dreams was at best a waste of time. More important, it would be an empathic break, analogous to asking a man in obvious pain if anything hurt.

Kohut did not use countertransference as a specific diagnostic tool. He regarded countertransference interferences in analysis as inevitable and urged an accepting realism regarding its presence. I had misunderstood the chapters on countertransferences to idealizing and mirroring transferences in *The Analysis of the Self* as a discussion in the spirit of Racker (1968), that is, that specific responses in the analyst could be used to understand the patient's psychology. This was not Kohut's view. He believed it was important to recognize countertransference interferences since these are likely to be the points where the analyst produces ruptures in the selfobject transference and, in this way, precipitates crucial issues in the analysis of self pathology. The analyst with a self-puntive attitude is likely to deny such breaches and repeat the patient's childhood traumata. The problem is not only that the selfobject fails the child. The failure is often denied and the legitimacy of the unmet needs ignored. But aside from insisting on this non-self-punitive attitude as necessary for analytic functioning, Kohut saw countertransference as an inevitable, important, but still objectionable part of psychoanalysis, without value of its own.

The Problem of Drive and Conflict Interpretation

With my patient, Kohut always regarded drive and conflict interpretations as inappropriate. At one point in the analysis, the patient complained of premature ejaculations. I wondered, to the patient, whether there was something about intercourse that made him anxious and want to finish quickly. The patient compliantly, but unfruitfully, explored this idea. Kohut pointed out that the interpretation, even if correct, was far from the patient's broad concerns. He thought that sexual arousal distressed the patient because he found it overstimulating. Similarly, when the patient engaged in a variety of exhibitionistic activities, culminating in an episode of intense erotic dancing before a group of friends, Kohut understood the material not in terms of phallic exhibitionism, but as an attempt by a threatened self to gain the environment's responsive mirroring. Empirically, Kohut's interpretation brought forth richer material from the patient than the interpretation of defense, anxiety, and drive-related motive.

As in most supervised analyses, supervision affected the analysis in complex ways. At the time I worked with Kohut, and especially in the context of this ''research analysis,'' I sometimes offered interpretations that were plausible within various theoretical frameworks but which I did not think were likely to be correct. I wanted, for example, to see if drive interpretations or interpretations about separation-individuation would be useful with this patient. Unfortunately, interpretations offered in this spirit are inevitably communicated differently from those the analyst thinks are most probably correct. They do not fairly test the validity of their content.

For Kohut, by the time he supervised me, such experiments were not so much scientifically invalid (he left this problem unaddressed in "The Two Analyses of Mr. Z.") as without real interest. The psychology of drives and their vicissitudes was part of psychoanalytic history for Kohut. Perhaps it required discussion until other analysts were properly educated, but these old ideas had no value to those who understood. I agree with Strozier (1985) that Kohut's position was not one of defensive arrogance but rather that of a brave, self-assured scientist convinced of the validity of his insights.

The Problem of Gratification

Much of the controversy surrounding Kohut's work centers on questions of "gratification." Some of the confusion arises from extensions of Kohut's work. In Models of the Mind, Gedo and Goldberg (1972) suggest that specific developmental pathology requires specific therapeutic interventions. A similar idea was put fourth earlier and in a different context by Anna Freud (1965) in Normality and Pathology in Childhood, but she was highly unspecific about the educational and psychotherapeutic interventions indicated for failures and arrests in development, although she recommended psychoanalysis for oedipal pathology. Gedo later elaborated the technical implications of the idea of varying the technique for various pathologies. Starting with Kohut's observation that disorders of the self are analyzable. Gedo (1976) enlarged the area of analyzable pathology and recommended specific approaches as essential in such analyses.

Kohut did not share the view that noninterpretative techniques should be used in analysis (see, for example, Gedo, 1976). In my experience, he was entirely "classical," in the sense that only interpretation was given to the patient. The difference was that demands for direct gratification were not generally interpreted as resistances to insight but rather as attempts, often legitimate, to receive needed supplies from the analyst. As noted earlier, the only exceptions to this position that Kohut described in his own practice were an instance in which he allowed a desperately frightened patient to hold his finger and the experimental scheduling of the hours of manic-depressive patients. Thus, Kohut concurred with my not visiting an exhibit in which my patient's work was shown and my not going to see the patient's apartment, which the patient thought would tell me much about him.

It was, however, appropriate to comment on the patient's disappointment and to view these requests not as resistance to verbalization but as attempts to let me know more, attempts with which, nonetheless, I was unwilling to cooperate.

Ordinary courtesy was the rule within sessions. Questions were to be answered or at least acknowledged. If the patient brought in photographs of his work, they were accepted.

Ideas on Self Psychology

Kohut often digressed to talk about self psychology and the reactions to it. Toward the end, he often spoke about his own illness. He said, more seriously than Strozier (1985) reports, that his administrative experiences in the American Psychoanalytic Association had led him to an interest in the developmental line of narcissism. He observed that the Association committees, composed largely of training analysts, presumably with good personal analytic experiences, functioned at least as badly as other committees, wasting vast amounts of time. He concluded that an important sector of the personality remained unanalyzed in many of these analysts. Since the problems that arose frequently reflected narcissistic issues, he thought this might well be the common unanalyzed area. (It would be fascinating to hear how other members of these committees experienced Kohut.)

As I already mentioned, by the time I worked with him Kohut was not particularly interested in the criticism of his work. Recall that on reading a particularly unfriendly review of *The Restoration of the Self*, his complaint was not about the disagreement but rather about the "stupidity" of the review. Kohut' s intellectual abilities and his education were first-rate by any standards. He was, I think, disappointed at the middle-brow level of much analytic discourse. Having worked hard to develop original ideas, he expected them to be considered seriously and treated with respect. It enraged him when they were rejected out of hand, with the voice of authority rather than scientific reason. The idea that his theories arose from a lack of appreciation of classical analytic concepts, patently false to anyone who has read his masterful description of its theories, particularly angered him. He reminded people that until his studies in narcissism he had been known as Mr. Psychoanalysis. If he deviated from the classical position, it was because he understood it well and because he appreciated the Freudian spirit of discovery.

The challenge left by Kohut is not to integrate self psychology into classical psychoanalysis; perhaps the two theories are simply incompatible. Rather, it involves the maintenance of an optimal dialogue among analysts of differing views. Self psychologists, starting with Kohut, want to go on with the development of their theories without forever having to reassert and rediscuss the foundation of their thinking. The emergence of a national self-psychological community, as manifest in the annual self psychology conferences and the series of volumes edited by Goldberg, attests to this need for independent development. At the same time, decreased dialogue between "classical" analysts and self psychologists would clearly be a loss for both groups.

Too often this dialogue is strained by informal assertions that self psychologists have lost their understanding of basic psychoanalytic concepts. Thus, for example, when Arnold Goldberg presented dream material in terms of self-state representations at a Regional Meeting of the Chicago Psychoanalytic Society and did not allude to the blatant erotic symbolism in the dream, he was chastised like a beginning candidate who had demonstrated his ignorance and resistance to unconscious sexual material rather than being treated as an experienced analyst whose failure to discuss this aspect of the material reflected a conscious and mature choice. Such certitude and assumptions that disagreement arises from ignorance and defect inevitably dulls scientific discourse. Kohut was discouraged by such responses to his work.[20]

DEATH AND MOURNING

During the time he supervised me, Kohut was chronically ill. His attitude toward his illness was characteristic—its symptoms fascinated him. I saw him for the last time during the winter of 1981, about seven months before his death. He was seeing some patients and supervisees at his home. I inquired about his health and was surprised by his detailed description of the muscle wasting in his legs and the effects

---

[20]Another recurring theme in this discussion is the position taken by such authors as Wallerstein (1985), who claim that it is unfortunate that Kohut formulated ideas antithetical to ego and drive psychology, thus dichotomizing the choice between self psychology and "classical" analysis. They feel that this interferes with the enrichment of analysis by Kohut's clinically valuable ideas and point out that it has long been understood that any psychological action is best understood from many viewpoints, that, indeed, according to the principle of multiple function, psychological acts are determined by many factors.

While this is a reasonable position for a clinician, it is precisely the sort of thing that interferes with the development of psychoanalysis as a science. Platt (1964) convincingly argues that sciences move forward best when sharply differentiable positions are tested against one another. Avoiding such distinct positions makes it impossible to design precise tests, which can clearly determine which position is accurate. As a result, the science does not move ahead.

of the exercise he was doing to try to relieve it. There was nothing hypochondriacal or self-pitying in this description. Nor was there any quality of denial or false optimism. Rather, this too was part of the always fascinating world, something to be examined and thought about. Vigorous, in his word, joyful, curiosity was so much part of Kohut's character that it continued even as he watched his own body deteriorate.

The appearance of *How Does Analysis Cure?* three years after Kohut's death, gave many of us an opportunity to continue the work of mourning. As I suspect occurred in many circles, a workshop of younger analysts, myself included, devoted almost a year to the careful study of this book. It clearly represents Kohut's thinking about psychoanalysis in the last years of his life, whether one likes those thoughts or not. The ideas in the book were no great surprise to anyone who knew and worked with Kohut. And this was something of a disappointment: we all secretly hoped the wizard's legacy would be a revelation.

With increasing analytic experience, my appreciation of Kohut's work has evolved. Although I believe I have a good ear for drive-related material and defenses, I am repeatedly impressed that most of my patients seem to be dealing with issues of regulating tension, failures to soothe themselves, or experiences of inner deadness and meaninglessness. Partly as a result of my supervisory experience with Kohut and the excellent outcome of the research analysis mentioned earlier, I take into analysis a broad range of patients. I therefore tend to see more analytic patients whose pathology does not center on conflict than analysts who attempt to avoid treating patients with central developmental deficits. Obviously, analysts who make evidence of a strongly engaged Oedipus complex a diagnostic prerequisite for undertaking analysis will confirm the impression that oedipal pathology is the major theme of most analyzable pathology.

At the same time, there are areas where I have found myself in growing disagreement with Kohut. These areas of disagreement are listed here for the purpose of exploring the psychology of myself as Kohut's student. No attempt is made to provide a balanced discussion of the issues themselves. The idea that the ultimate explanation of mental life is not to be found in the vissicitudes of libidinal and aggressive drives was often accompanied in Kohut's discourse by a lack of specificity and concreteness in discussions of early development. Abstract, ethereal "feeling states" and gleams in maternal eyes seemed to replace the concrete, rather gross experiences in which life is lived. As I watched my own children grow up, listened to my patients (and at times, with child patients, observed their parents), and taught courses in early development based on observation, I found that formative experiences were usually not in the least subtle. Rather, they were quite flagrant, if only one allowed oneself to see them. For example, Kohut often discussed "latent parental psychoses." These psychoses seem to me to be latent only in the sense that they have not been formally diagnosed and that they are covered in public to the extent that people who want to deny their presence can do so without seeming crazy themselves.

With regard to Kohut's description of vague "feeling states," I doubt that inchoate feeling states remain that way for long, except in certain rare pathologies. Instead, they find symbolic expression, which in turn leads to attempts to solve the problem through manipulations of the symbols. Kohut was, I think, getting at this idea in his discussion of the sexualization of narcissistic needs. But attempting to counteract the undue attention to the details of these symbolic phenomena and their easy confusion with the vicissitudes of drives, Kohut paid little attention to the issue of symbol formation and the development of symbolic processes. Melanie Klein's detailed discussion of these matters seems to me potentially and usefully integratable with Kohut's work. In any case, the disparagement of detailed study of the workings of fantasy processes, in favor of attention to the overall feeling state represented in the fantasy seems to me now to be an error, both in theory and analytic practice.[21]

Another area of disagreement lies in the goal of analytic work as expressed by Kohut in the first chapter of *The Restoration of the Self* and later in *How Does Analysis Cure?* I have no argument with the pragmatic assertion that some patients are satisfied with analyses that while clearly incomplete leave them more productive, creative, and alive to the world than they were. Nor do I disagree with the idea that there are situations where discretion is the better part of valor and that certain experiences are wisely left unexplored with some patients. But such pragmatic considerations should be treated for what they are—partial failures of the analytic process. Furthermore, I am skeptical that solu-

---

[21]A colleague tells the following story of Kohut as a candidate. Kohut was presenting a case in a seminar and observed that the patient's associations clearly referred to Kohut's recent marriage. Kohut was perplexed. He had not told the patient of his marriage, nor was it likely that the patient would have heard of the marriage from other sources. As he spoke, he drummed the fingers of his left hand against his forehead, displaying his wedding ring. This episode and the incident I described earlier of Kohut's inaccurate description of the "little piggy" game, as well as his customary indifference to the details of dream content and fantasy, suggest to me that Kohut's distaste for highly elaborate, detectivelike investigations, of which some analysts are so proud, originated in part in a cognitive style that did not involve detailed attention to external evidence as a major source of information.

tions to life's problems that ignore important aspects of the individual's biology can really be very satisfactory.

While there may be patients with generally satisfactory results who do not engage in self-analysis following treatment, I see these patients as being left without the major benefit of analysis—the capacity for continued development. Here I am not referring primarily to conscious self-analytic work, which, as Weiss (1981) has observed, is often nothing more than obsessional rumination. Rather, I mean the unconscious and preconscious process of continued working over, which I have postulated to be central to mental health in general and development in particular (Galatzer-Levy, in press).

Related to this area of disagreement is Kohut's view, which though looser is essentially in accord with classical views—that people have a nuclear program of development set at birth or shortly thereafter, and that pathology is the failure to realize some version or substitute for this program. While I think there are such programs, I believe they constitute only a portion of the developmental task. I see one of the central tasks of normal development as the creation of new programs for oneself.

The problem of the general presence of guilt and its centrality in human psychology is not, to my mind, adequately solved by the assumption of a very common but nonetheless pathological configuration in psychological development.

Finally, I disagree vigorously with Kohut's denigration of psychoanalytically informed infant research as a source of information useful to the analyst. While this research can (and does) go astray by replacing descriptions of internal experience with descriptions of social interaction, these studies are of the greatest value both to the analytic theorist and the clinician in understanding early development. Just as the work of art (Trosman, 1985) can teach the analytic reader about psychology despite its limits as an incomplete and artistically contrived account, so too can behavioral accounts of infant development help the analyst to understand people.

I mention these areas of substantial disagreement to illustrate a process of an intellectual transmuting internalization. As parts of Kohut's work become increasingly my own, they become separated from the personality of their creator. Other parts of his work are discarded. Similarly, Kohut's deep enthusiasm for psychoanalysis and psychoanalytic investigation is transformed and joins the many other sources of a similar enthusiasm in myself.

During the last two years, as part of a paper on the analysis of manic-depressive patients, I have presented some of the material from the analysis for which Kohut served as consultant. The paper has generally been well received. In it I assume many of the findings of self psychology, but my major points are not really part of a self psychology framework. In fact, as I mentioned earlier, Kohut himself did not find my first formulations of these ideas particularly interesting.

This does not keep me from being labeled a "Kohutian." Like many of his students, I want both to hold onto what Kohut taught me and not be constrained by his work. I was dismayed that labeling became so important. When I first presented my analytic work with manic-depressive patients at the research seminar of the Institute, a deeply admired former teacher said sadly, "So, you've become a Kohutian!" I never intended to join a camp, but rather to present what I had learned and inferred from my clinical work. I wanted to quote another respected colleague who, when asked if he was Kohutian or "classical" responded, "Neither, I'm a psychoanalyst." The sense that an appreciation of Kohut' s work alienates one from significant numbers of (especially older) analysts saddens me.

It is odd how, even in Chicago, Kohut' s ideas continue to carry with them, for some analysts, the mark of heresy. I am not referring here to scientific disagreement, however vigorous and even personalized, but rather to a notion that analysts who concur with Kohut's ideas have set themselves apart and are in some sort of danger. The danger is one of being led astray from the "truth" and leading others astray. Recently, when an analyst gave a thorough and scholarly discussion of the development of female sexuality from a self psychology point of view, a friend commented to me that the analyst "had come out of the closet." Not infrequently, when I teach in the various programs at the analytic institute, discussing material from several viewpoints, students will ask, in a conspiratorial tone, what I really think. Their manner often suggests that we are all Marranos. It may be safe to express our Kohutian ideas among ourselves, but we must be cautious lest the authorities hear what we think.

Miller (1985) notes the curiosity of analysts and candidates about "how Kohut actually worked." He attributes this curiosity to the scattered nature of Kohut's remarks on technique and describes his experience of consultation with Kohut. As with my own experience, there was no inconsistency between Kohut's public statements and what he told Miller. Both my experience with Kohut and the experience of being asked about the consultation are like Miller's in this regard, but I understand the curiosity differently. There is clearly a fantasy, sometimes expressed openly, that Kohut secretly advocated techniques that departed significantly from those of classical analysis. It is common to hear that the burdensome metapsychological explanations in *The Analysis of the Self* are there for political reasons. In essence Kohut is seen as a (perhaps false) messiah to whom a few of us had access and whose secret doctrines and practices we may reveal. According to this fantasy, as with other messiahs, the full extent of his doctrines and the assertion of his position as the messiah have to be introduced with caution so as not to unduly disrupt the world.[22]

Perhaps one source for these ideas is the discrepancy between Freud's written descriptions of his technique and what Freud actually did with his patients. For better or worse, it is clear now that Freud was not a "classical" analyst, and it is tempting to think that knowing what the "master" actually did would be useful (especially for rationalizing one's own behavior or denigating his). With Kohut, given his emphasis on patients' "needs" as opposed to their "wishes," it seems to many that he must have gratified those "needs" or—what amounts to the same thing—encouraged the illusion of gratification.

I think we are dealing here with the vicissitudes of idealization and envy. A notion that supports idealization is that despite the limitations and failings suggested by Kohut's writings, additional, secret information is available, that will reveal Kohut's profound wisdom and miraculous abilities to deal with difficult problems. Also connected to idealization is the idea that more information will allow the listener to become more like Kohut. Occasionally one has the experience that just having made contact with someone who knew Kohut, independent of what is said, produces a sense of magical relatedness and potential merger with the idealized leader. One is treated like someone who has seen a miracle.

On the other side, material about what Kohut actually said is sometimes elicited in a spirit of destructive envy. Such questions often take the form of attempts to find evidence that Kohut's technique was not "pure," that he recommended or practiced techniques that put him beyond the analytic pale. This quality of being ready to spring at some supposed fault in Kohut's work is clearly aimed at spoiling and befouling his image.

The analytic community is very familiar with such activities. A large literature about Freud centers on similar ideas that he was a master each one of whose actions carried a lesson for the admiring student.

---

[22]This image is messianic in the sense that the leader is seen as the voice of a higher power—in this instance psychoanalytic truth.

The similarities of the response to Kohut in psychoanalysis to responses to messianic ideas within Judaism are remarkable. These include the belief that truth is embodied in an individual, that there is great danger from a false messiah, that the messiah will only gradually reveal himself, that he will be surrounded by followers (faithful and unfaithful), that his every act is of significance, that his validity is to be examined in the light of canonical texts and that lessons in the avoidance of false messiahs are to be learned through the study of past messianic heresy (Scholem, 1957, 1971).

Alternatively, secret, conspiratorially hidden information will reveal the basic flaw in everything he did and bring it toppling to the ground. Such attitudes are also familiar from other contexts, most notably religious situations, in which masters and teachers are seen as embodying great wisdom in their every act. In the Talmud, for example, Rabbi Akiva reports following his teacher to the outhouse, where he learned five important things (Finkelstein, 1936).

A variation on this theme is the tendency to displace some of the negative feeling from the leader to his students. Occasionally one hears responses to Kohut from his contemporaries that transparently reflect resentment that all their vigorous efforts did not result in the major creative developments Kohut made. And it is common to hear hostile remarks about close students of Kohut who "misunderstood" and perverted Kohut's teaching.

For all its discomforts, we have an opportunity with Kohut's ideas to study the vicissitudes of idealization and envy within a scientific community. Steiner (1985) asserts that "controversial" discussions between the Kleinian and the classical members of the British psychoanalytic association were successful, in the sense that useful dialogue continued between the two groups, scientific ideas were clarified, and the British Society's work of training analysts and supporting analytic development continued despite strong emotional disagreement and intense personal feeling. He argues that the discussions were successful, in part, because of their congruence with their content—that precisely because the discussions concerned primitive emotional states, it became possible to partly work through these emotional states as they occurred in the groups and individuals involved in the discussions. Along these lines, it is reasonable to expect that the fact that we are discussing the vicissitudes of narcissism will be most helpful in working through the narcissistic issues involved in the process of discussion.

CONCLUSION

I do not want to join the seemingly endless discussion of what Thomas Kuhn "really" means by a "scientific revolution" or a "paradigm" as applied to psychoanalysis. My reading of his work leads me to be further interested in the psychology of practicing scientists and to believe that such psychological issues are of importance to the philosopher and historian of science. I have tried to present here, in relatively uncensored form, some of the qualities of the experience of being involved in a community as a major new model for thinking about phenomena emerged. It is clearly impossible to separate the personal experience and development from the evolution of my scientific thought. During the period described in this paper, I moved from being a beginning student of psychiatry to becoming a teacher of psychiatrists and analysts. I had a personal analysis, which included extensive examination of the vicissitudes of narcissism; married and had four children. I also treated many patients using psychotherapy and psychoanalysis, read widely, and had the untold life experiences one might expect in the 15 years between my 26th and the 41st year. It would be foolhardy to try to separate these developments from the gradual working over of intellectual and practical ideas that led from my surprise at discovering that Kohut was not physically large to a valuing and making my own of some of his ideas and ideals. The realities of an individual's development are simply too complex to say, "Here we see clearly how exposure to Kohut affected him."

Yet, I think my experience is, in important ways, far from unique. Many colleagues who highly value Kohut's contributions have unconflictedly gone on to explore realms and viewpoints that Kohut would have found of little interest. People who have worked with self psychology issues over an extended period of time vary in their current positions, from seeing self psychology as the dominant paradigm with which they understand psychoanalytic data, to a sense that it is sometimes useful. Nonetheless, each of these positions seems to be accompanied by an increased specificity in what is accepted and rejected, a separation of ideas and attitudes from the person of Kohut, a decreased stridency of outlook, and transformations and developments of the ideas and ideals so as to integrate them with the rest of the personality and interests of the analyst.

In his composite portrait of an early 20th-century physicist who resisted the emerging new physics, Russell McCorrmach (1982) shows the despair and confusion that arise when a "normal science," which ordered the world, passes into history and leaves the scientist unsupported by a coherent world view. McCorrmach's book is particularly valuable because it integrates a description of individual psychology with the historical situation, testifying to the complex interrelationship between the emotional and intellectual life of the scientist.

Oddly, while writers interested in psychoanalysis have attended to Kuhn's ideas about paradigms and scientific revolutions from an inappropriately prescriptive point of view (Knight, 1985), they have not explored the psychology of the phenomena so vividly described by Kuhn (1964). One of the difficulties with Kuhn's idea of a paradigm, as he himself confirms, (Kuhn, 1974), is the multiplicity of meanings he gives it. Careful dissection of Kuhn's use of this term yields a logically clarifying list of his meanings. Yet, when so clear a thinker as Kuhn appears so confused, we must suspect that the concepts he has lumped together must be intimately related, in some as yet to be specified way.

The reader of this paper must be impressed that it describes a transmuting internalization of an idealized figure. What began as a gross idealization led, through a series of nontraumatic disappointments, to increasingly selective identifications with aspects of Kohut's personality, values, and ideas appropriate to my developmental needs as a young analyst. Except in an artificial and antipsychological way, it would be impossible to separate the contents of these internalizations— to argue, say, that my readiness to value Kohut's intellectual contribution could have been independent of my response to his charismatic style.

I think that very similar processes must go on in the lives of many scientists, although perhaps not so self-consciously and often not in nearly so nontraumatic a fashion. The several types of paradigms first lumped together and then dissected by Kuhn and his co-workers can be understood as representing the various stages of a process of transmuting internalization of an (often personified) scientific ideal. For approximately 200 years, physics was associated with the person of Isaac Newton, whose authority was sufficient to impede the development of various aspects of that science in important areas such as optics. More immediately, psychoanalysis remains closely linked to the person of Freud; and various developments of psychoanalysis, including self psychology, remain associated with the person of their founders. Sometimes these associations are exploited in confused attacks on disciplines; sometimes they are used in support of authoritative positions; sometimes they lead to irrational overvaluation of anything associated with the idealized founder and other related phenomena.

In this light, the material described in this paper is a contribution to the intrapsychic description of the situation that Kuhn described sociologically and historically as paradigm formation. The "disciplinary matrix" Kuhn describes as embodied in "scientific communities" is the selfobject function of those communities for their members. Abstract ideas cannot be supported in a matrix (or anything else); only the people having those ideas can be supported.

REFERENCES

Finkelstein, B. (1936), *Akiva*. Jewish Publication Society.

Freiden, R., Levy, R. & Harmon, R. (1970), A student-community planned health project for the poor. *New England Journal of Medicine*, 283:1142–1157.

Freud, A. (1965), *Normality and Pathology in Childhood*. New York: International Universities Press.

Galatzer-Levy, R. (1982), On the opening phase of the treatment of hypochondriasis. *Internat. J. Psychother.*

_____ (in press), On working through: A model from artificial intelligence. *J. Amer. Psychoanal. Assn.*

_____ (1987), Manic-depressive illness: Analytic experience and a hypothesis. In: *Frontiers in Self Psychology*, ed. A. Goldberg. Hillsdale, NJ: The Analytic Press, 87–102.

Gedo, J. (1976). *Beyond Interpretation*. New York: International Universities Press.

_____ & Goldberg, A. (1972), *Models of the Mind*. Chicago: University of Chicago Press.

Knight, I. (1985), Paradigms and crises in psychoanalysis. *Psychoanal. Quart.*, 54:597–614.

Kohut, H. (1971), *The Analysis of the Self*. New York: International Universities Press.

_____ (1976), *The Restoration of the Self*. New York: International Universities Press.

Kuhn, T. (1964), *The Structure of Scientific Revolutions*. Chicago: University of Chicago Press.

_____ (1974), Second thoughts on paradigms. In: *The Structure of Sientific Theories*, ed. F. Suppe. Urbana: University of Illinois Press.

Levy, R. (1973), Untoward effects of drug education. *Amer. J. Public Health*, 63:1071–1073.

_____ (1974), Analysis of calls to a drug-crisis intervention service. *J. Psychedelic Drugs*, 6:143–152.

_____ & Brown, A. R. (1971), A drug crisis intervention unit: Analysis of the first year of operation. (Abst.) *Clin. Research*, 19:502.

_____ & Halikas, J. (1972), Illicit pentazocine (Talwin) use: A report of thirteen cases. *Internat. J. Addiction*, 7:693–700.

Little, M. (1985), Winnicott working in areas where psychotic anxieties predominate. *Free Associations*, 3:9–42.

Mach, E. (1980), *Great Pianists Speak for Themselves*. New York: Dodd Mead.

McCorrmach, R. (1982), *Night Thoughts of a Classical Physicist*. Cambridge, MA: Harvard University Press.

Miller, J. (1985), How Kohut actually worked. In: *Advances in Self Psychology*, Vol. 1, ed. A. Goldberg. pp. 13–30. New York: Guilford.

Offenkrantz, W. & Tobin, A. (1975), Short term psychotherapy. In: *American Handbook of Psychiatry*, S. Arieti, ed. New York: Basic Books.

Platt, J. R. (1964), Strong inference. *Science*, 146:347–353.

Racker, H. (1968), *Transference and Countertransference*. New York: International Universities Press.

Schafer, R. (1964), *Aspects of Internalization*. New York: International Universities Press.

Schnabel, A. (1942), *Music and the Line of Most Resistance*. New York: De Capo Press, 1969.

Scholem, G. (1957), *Sabbatai Sevi: The Mystical Messiah* (trans. R. Weblowsky). Princeton, NJ: Princeton University Press, 1973.

_____ (1971), *The Messianic Idea in Judaism and Other Essays on Jewish Spirituality*. New York: Schocken.

Steiner, R. (1985), Some thoughts about tradition and change arising from an examination of the British Psychoanalytic Society's controversial discussion (1943–1944). *Internat. Rev. Psychoanal.*, 12:27–72.

Stolorow, R. & Atwood, G., (1979), *Faces in a Cloud*. New York: Aronson.

Strozier, C. (1985), Glimpses of a life: Heinz Kohut (1913–1981. In: A. Goldberg, ed., *Advances in Self Psychology*, Vol. 1. New York: Guilford.

Sullivan, H. S. (1962), *Schizophrenia as a Human Process*. New York: Norton.

Trosman, H. (1985), *Freud and the Imaginative World*. Hillsdale, NJ: The Analytic Press.

Wallerstein, R. (1976), Psychoanalysis as a science: Its present status and its future tasks. *Psychol. Issues,* 9:198–228.

_____ (1985), How does self psychology differ in practice? *Internat. J. Psychoanal.,* 66:391–404.

Weiss, S. (1981), Reflections on the psychoanalytic process, with special emphasis on child analysis and self-analysis. *The Annual of Psychoanalysis,* 9:43–56. New York: International Universities Press.

Chapter 2

On Supervision with Heinz Kohut

Sheldon J. Meyers

This paper is about my experience with Heinz Kohut as a supervisor and as a teacher. It is an attempt to convey how this experience both affected me as a person and contributed to my development as a psychoanalyst. The paper describes the experience and the thoughts it stimulated, and is interspersed with descriptions of the consultation and clinical material. I first met Heinz Kohut for my matriculation interviews at the Institute for Psychoanalysis in Chicago in 1968. Later, as an advanced candidate, I was again exposed to Kohut at the Institute. Although he was not teaching a regular course at that time, he gave several lectures in the self psychology course. Kohut was a very charismatic teacher. He had an exquisite grasp of clinical material and an extraordinary ability to articulate it. He was able to engage people in listening to how he experienced another person and to how he technically would deal with that person in treatment. He presented and discussed very difficult cases utilizing his new theories, and the candidates responded to him with respect and admiration. An intellectual fervor surrounded him at that time. I found his new theories useful, helpful, and exciting, particularly with those patients who were unresponsive to a classical approach.

Soon after graduating from the Institute in 1975, I was invited to attend a postgraduate workshop on self psychology led by Kohut. I eventually became the workshop's secretary for two years and in this capacity got to know Kohut in a more personal way. The workshop met monthly and was regularly attended by people coming from various parts of the United States, Canada, and, occasionally, Europe. Perhaps we in Chicago took for granted this man who flourished in such a creative way and who attracted bright people from all over the country. Kohut always spoke spontaneously to the issue at hand. He shared his reactions to clinical material in sensitive and experiential terms. The workshop was composed of many bright, intellectual, young analysts who provided a stimulating and responsive environment for Kohut and his new ideas.

Some of the analysts who came to the workshop from other parts of the country saw Kohut in supervision. I thought it would be a wonderful educational experience to be supervised by him. Most people who had been supervised by Kohut in Chicago had been supervised at an earlier time, often as part of their curriculum at the Institute. I was not sure that he would accept me for supervision, he seemed to be only seeing out-of-town people.

Although I had extensively read the self-psychology literature, my understanding had been skewed by my education and personal analysis. To gain a better understanding, I wanted to be supervised by Kohut. I contacted him in November of 1978 and began consultation with him once a month until July 1981. He died three months later in October 1981.[1] Rather than taking detailed notes of our sessions, I relied on experiencing the process in order to integrate what I had learned. Illness or vacations sometimes interrupted our consultations for as long as three months. We usually met in Kohut's office at the Institute, but while he was recuperating from illness, I saw him in his study at his home. He seemed more relaxed in his home, probably because he could be more informal and less professional than in his office. In general, he was congenial, friendly and put me at ease quickly. He appeared to be open to me and my ideas. Yet he was always the consummate teacher, attempting to illustrate his theories and ideas from clinical material. He sat in a hard-backed, wooden chair that seemed stiff and austere, although he was very informal and loose in his body language. He listened carefully to the material presented to him, often appearing lost in thought. At times, with a slight smile on his face, he seemed to relish certain material that was focal to teaching me something of his viewpoint. He made it very clear that this was what he wanted to do in the consulting process rather than to supervise or to help me manage a case directly.

My overall feeling was that he was a superb clinician who followed

---

[1]This was the exact time that Jule Miller consulted with Kohut. See his excellent report of his experience (Miller, 1985).

the material and understood it from the surface down. Initially his technique surprised me by being very classical. He believed that a positive transference needed to be established before one could begin to interpret and explain the transference that existed. He felt this was best facilitated by understanding the patient's affect state and conveying that understanding to him. Strikingly, Kohut operated by utilizing clinical theory long familiar to all psychoanalysts. His notions of selfobject transferences, however, were metapsychologically different from the classical theory of instincts and defenses. The instincts and defenses were dealt with as secondary elaborations of failed selfobject relationships. Because his notions departed from classical metapsychology, his clinical stance was easily misunderstood by some analysts and thought to be nonanalytic. Kohut's definition of transference was more encompassing than transference of drive and defense, but his technique was psychoanalytic. He stated that the analyst needed to establish a positive transference configuration in the analytic situation, and then it could be interpreted in its positive or negative forms. This would lead to internalization, which strengthened strucure and which then could endure in more mature forms. He believed that these transferences should first be interpreted in the here and now of the analytic situation and then linked to the genetic precursors as explanations. With the strengthening of the self-structure and with the subsequent decrease of drive intensity, conflicts over libidinal and aggressive drives could be managed more easily by the patient. This was particularly true of the narcissistic personality disorders but could be applied to higher developmental pathology.

The first case that I discussed with Kohut was that of a 45-year-old male lawyer who appeared to be very bright, had a very conflicted marriage, worked very hard professionally, and had high expectations of success in his field. He was depressed and felt as if he were getting nowhere in life. The patient was very reluctant to engage in the analysis, being very resistant to looking at the analytic relationship. He had an intense fear of being hurt if his relationship with me became too important to him.

He had a cold, distant, hypochondriacal mother and an infantile, competitive father whom he could never please. His depression seemed related to unfulfilled longings for women to respond to and love him, and for older, powerful, men to admire him. He was charming and engaging but he had difficulty sustaining important relationships as his needs were difficult to satisfy. I found this patient very resistant, and I was unable to engage him in the analytic process. The patient was intensely self-occupied, finding it difficult to experience another person as separate. For a long time there were conflicts over scheduled hours and missed appointments, signifying that the analysis and the analyst were unimportant items on his agenda.

I presented this case to Kohut because I felt it represented the type of patient who was so easily injured narcissistically that there was a reluctance to engage in treatment. Kohut listened very carefully and felt that my view of looking at the patient as resistant was interfering with the analytic process. He said that the patient was engaging in treatment in the way that he needed. This was the transference that needed to be established, rather than interpreted as resistance. My preconceived theoretical notion of resistance to the analytic relationship got in the way of the process. He said, "When the patient exhibits anger toward you, you cannot interpret it as transference this early in the relationship. He experiences the anger as real, and it needs to come out in the analysis and be accepted." It is often thought that Kohut did not deal with angry transferences at any level, because the gratification of selfobject needs precluded anger in the analysis. This was not true in my experience. These early consulting sesssions with Kohut made me aware that I was using analytic technique based on learned formulae that had interfered with my following the process with this patient who was "resistant." According to Kohut, the patient was looking for, but frightened of, "a good relationship with a man he could look up to in order to feel good about himself." He was searching for a good father–son relationship. My focusing on his resistance and on his anger toward me for not allowing him to change appointments fell on deaf ears.

Kohut used this case to point out that to establish a transference, the patient needs to feel understood and accepted at the level of his interaction in the here and now. The patient's anger and fear of engaging me was over not being recognized and accepted for himself. He experienced my "classical stance" as cold, controlling, and distancing, as his parents had been. Repeated interpretations to him about the transference as resistance had no apparent effect; reality for him was no different from his original genetic experience. The consultation centered on listening and understanding the patient from the surface down. I was repeatedly told not to make theoretical assumptions, but to listen to the patient, to myself, and to the process. As I was better able to grasp this idea and as I began to deal with the patient more in the process than in theory, the analytic material began to shift. The patient turned to me as the father he had never had in order to deal with the upsetting, unfulfilling experiences he had with his mother, his wife, and women in general.

Kohut also felt that I was interpreting dreams too much in terms of very specific impulses and defenses. He suggested that they should be viewed as broad reconstructions of what the patient felt as a child and what was being revived in the treatment with me now in the transference. This is not to say that later on in the treatment a more specific reconstruction would not be indicated. For example, the patient presented a dream in the second month of treatment about a pig being born: "I had a bizarre dream about a woman giving birth to a baby that was a pig. At the delivery, this baby [pig] needed to be resuscitated. I cut the head off the pig and began to resuscitate it. I got frightened. Why did I cut the head off?" His associations were that it "was a crazy, bizarre dream. The pig popped out. It was something horrible and frightening. I felt I was doing something crazy." I said, "The pig represented something very disturbing inside of you that you feel you can't handle appropriately once it pops out." He further associated to a girl he had dated who became psychotic and whom he had left, thus not helping her. I pointed out that he was talking about the angry bizarre things inside of him that he felt he could not handle if they came out.

Kohut felt that the interpretation of this dream this early was too specific to the defended impulse and should be more general, having to do with the sense of himself as the pig, a devaluation of his mother, and the sordid, horrible world in which he grew up. Kohut encouraged me to make broad empathic statements about the here and now when the patient seemed reluctant to be involved with me. He also suggested that the patient be told, in an empathic way, that it was difficult for him to acknowledge his need for another person because of what he missed from both of his parents. These kind of interventions did decrease the patient's "resistance" to his involvement in the analytic process. The patient did not feel criticized and was able to engage me in a more genuine and positive way.

These consultations with Kohut were extremely helpful to me in dealing with a sensitive, difficult patient who initially had a great deal of trouble acknowledging my importance to him. He could engage in the treatment only after he began to feel safe because he felt understood and accepted. Classical technique employing resistance analysis with this person with narcissistic vulnerability only created iatrogenic anger and resistance to my interventions. Kohut's technique was psychoanalytic. Empathy and conveying what the patient was experiencing was crucial before interpretation, explanation, and reconstruction could take place. Freud (1913) stated that transference should not be interpreted

> until an effective transference has been established in the patient, a proper rapport with him. It remains the first aim of treatment to attach him to

it and to the person of the doctor. To insure this nothing need be done but to give him time. If one exhibits a serious interest in him, . . . he will of himself form such an attachment and link the doctor up with one of the imagos of the people by whom he was accustomed to be treated with affection. It is certainly possible to forfeit this first success if from the start one takes up any standpoint other than one of sympathetic understanding, such as a moralizing one, or . . . like . . . a contending party [like a parent or a spouse] [p.139–140].

Freud indicated that the patient needed an atmosphere of understanding and helpfulness that would facilitate the positive and unobjectionable transference if the analytic transference was to be established and then analyzed. The fact that Kohut was classical in his technique was very surprising to me because there was no hint of it in his early writings, which never described how he worked technically with patients. I suspect he felt that analysts would use classical technique incorporating his new concept of selfobject transferences. In 1979, in a panel on the Bipolar Self at the American Psychoanalytic Association, he extensively described his clinical technique as psychoanalytic. His technique was acknowledged as classical by both Michael Basch and Robert Wallerstein, who were on that panel (Meyers, 1981). Kohut (1984) stated that ''self psychology relies on the same tools as traditional analysis (interpretation followed by working through in an atmosphere of abstinences) to bring about the analytic cure . . .'' (p. 75).

In reflecting on this case, I feel that Kohut engaged me in a parallel process in the supervisory alliance (Fleming and Benedek, 1966). He was accepting of me and understanding of my disagreements with him. He tried to show me the greater explanatory power of his theory for understanding the patient. His sensitivity to my feelings were paramount even though he pointed out faults, errors, and mistakes. His criticisms were helpful and could be integrated because of his accepting and understanding attitude. He seemed to enjoy the consultative process. He would take summary notes after the supervisory session and read them out loud to me at the beginning of our next session. This served as a good review for his sense of the process. More important, it was a way of airing our differences of opinion and constructive criticism in an open, collegial way. It impressed me that his empathic position seemed to be equidistant between me and the patient. He was therefore able to convey to me what the patient was experiencing in a way I could grasp without defensiveness.

Kohut's empathic responses were not infallible. At times I felt that his use of empathy was forced and not necessarily on target. One of those times I recall vividly occurred when I had gotten caught in the rain before going to my consultation with Kohut. He saw that I was wet, solicitously inquired about my comfort, and wondered if I wanted to put on a dry suit. He kept one in his closet in case he ever got caught in the rain, and he generously offered it to me. I was pleased by the offer. But then I looked at Kohut, sitting across from me forty pounds lighter than I; he was already showing signs of his chronic illness. I sat there with a broad grin, which he questioned. I thanked him for his offer and, noting our size difference, declined. He laughed and said, "Of course," and we started to work. This incident made me realize that his desire to be empathic sometimes was automatic. Nonetheless, this experience made Kohut more human, less ideal, and it enhanced our working alliance.

After I had been working with Kohut for about a year, he referred a patient to me whom he had seen in diagnostic consultation. The patient was a 32-year-old, large, powerful looking man, a librarian. He had a distant relationship with his wife of three years. Through his life, he had had difficulty sustaining involved relationships with women but had several good male friends. The patient had recently been narcissistically injured by his boss, an older man, whom he admired and greatly idealized. His boss had angrily criticized and fired the patient. He was crushed, humiliated, and came to me feeling very anxious, angry, and vulnerable. In the first interview he felt quite upset and felt that I looked too young to help him, that he wanted an older more experienced analyst. He saw me as neither understanding nor helpful and could not understand how Kohut could have made the referral. He assumed I would start treating him immediately and was upset that I was attempting to evaluate him diagnostically. I had doubts about whether I could analyze this patient. But because Kohut had referred this patient and was available for consultation, I accepted the patient for analysis after consulting with Kohut, who felt the man was analyzable.

I was upset by the patient's confrontational, attacking attitude at the start of treatment. There was very little that I could do right. A therapeutic alliance did not exist. Kohut patiently attempted to get me to make broad statements in the here and now rather than pursuing the details of free association and looking for the vicissitudes of transference and resistance. He felt that the details I sought could be brought in at a later date. The questions I asked in an attempt to calm my own anxiety were not helpful to the patient. Kohut emphasized the crucial importance of the analytic stance and capacity to listen, especially in the initial phase of analysis. He tried to dissuade me from interpreting resistance as transference. Such interpretation was very crucial to me because I felt beleaguered by the constant attacks of this patient, and to protect myself I defensively interpreted the patient's "acted-in" anger as transference.

The patient heard my interpretations as saying to him that he was not justified in being angry (with me) and that he was at fault as I was not doing anything wrong. He felt attacked and insisted that I acknowledge that I was injuring him. He said, "You analysts always think you are right." Kohut insisted that if the proper attitude of understanding and accepting is communicated over a long enough period of time, the patient will begin to be less fearful of analytic involvement. The patient's intense attacks on me continued for several months. Kohut suggested that I try to understand the patient's predicament. He said, "How terrible it felt for him to be dropped by someone who was so important to him and how angry he obviously was." Kohut emphasized that when anger was displaced onto me from the person who had hurt the patient, I recognize it as transference anger and not take it personally. The analyst must accept the anger without retreating, without acting it out in retaliation, or without attempting to interpret it as transference or as a defense in order to distance himself from it.

Kohut felt it was a mistake to interpret anger as transference or as resistance until a sufficiently solid relationship was established. This was not to avoid the anger or to gratify the patient. It was to facilitate the interpretation of anger later on in the context of a transference interaction, where it could be dealt with analytically. This was clearly a psychoanalytic stance. This patient in particular, Kohut insisted, was so upset that he needed to feel that I was trying to understand and to be helpful to him. Without this basis for a relationship, there could be no transference relationship to interpret later. I think this aspect of Kohut's theory and technique is often misunderstood. Kohut is often criticized for not dealing with or interpreting anger. It is claimed that Kohut's position was that if the analyst "gratified" the patient in the selfobject transference, the anger would disappear. This could not be a more misperceived sense of how Kohut worked. He knew that anger needed to be dealt with, pointed out, and interpreted after the relationship had developed sufficiently so that when the patient felt "injured" in the transference he could accept his angry responses and see that he was responding to something from his more infantile "self" in terms of the selfobject transference.

Anger was constantly the focal point and "acted in" in the process with this easily injured patient. The patient would often storm from the room when hurt. This anger directed at me became easier for me to accept because of the supervisory relationship. Kohut saw the patient's anger positively, as a way of controlling his environment and feeling effective. The patient needed to recognize that he felt helpless and ineffective because he had been humiliated and injured by his boss. His anger was secondary to this injury and not due to primary sadism. Gradually, the positive therapeutic relationship and selfobject transference began to emerge when the patient reluctantly admitted that I was more available to him than his ex-boss, whom he still admired.

Kohut believed the primary pathology in this case was due to a father who did not rescue this man from his problems with a mother who was emotionallly unavailable and unable to experience her son's separateness. The mother was an inept, inadequate woman who was ''under her husband's thumb.'' The father was a very powerful, idealized, and yet totally unempathic person who clearly did not see his son as separate from himself. He often lost control and sadistically berated the patient for his disappointing behavior and was virulently critical of him. It was this identification with the father that the patient often acted out with me. Clinically the positive transference felt more maternal than paternal to me. Kohut disagreed with this assessment and said the pathology in this case was cearly due to the father, as it was in the Schreber case (Freud, 1911).

Kohut was very interested in my case and said that it needed to be published, as most cases in the self psychology literature demonstrated pathological involvement with the mother. I felt that judgment to be premature, given the clinical ''gut'' feeling I had of the transference. I tried to accept and understand what Kohut postulated but found it difficult in the face of contrary clinical evidence. That he felt so convinced without adequate clinical confirmation led to some disillusionment on my part. I thought that he was not following his cardinal rule not to be influenced by (experience-distant) theory but rather to follow the process (experience-near). This difference of opinion heightened the importance of following the experience-near aspect of the case. I idealized Kohut less and was disquieted at first by disagreeing with him. Freud (1912) stated that the technique required for research, opposes the one required for treatment. ''Cases which are devoted from the first to scientific purposes and are treated accordingly suffer in their outcome; while the most successful cases are those which one proceeds . . . without any purpose in view, allows oneself to be taken by surprise by any new turn in them, and always meets them with an open mind, free from any presuppositions'' (p. 114). It was clear that Freud was speaking of an experience-near approach taking precedence over experience-distant theory.

Kohut and I agreed to put aside our differences and follow the process to see which way the patient would lead us. I could see

Kohut's desire to gather evidence for publication of an important case with primary paternal involvement in the pathology. In spite of his own desire, he listened to me, as the analyst, experiencing the material and following it without premature closure. I thought that the patient was holding on to his fantasized idealized relationship with his ex-boss to avoid involvement with me. Kohut said no, that he was involved in a massive transference reaction to the other man and that it would fade as his involvement with me increased. I needed to be accepting, empathic, and understanding. This was difficult for me to accept as I believed the "defenses" were so fixed and intense. Gradually, however, I began to realize that the patient and I were working together toward a common goal. We were gradually developing a working alliance. As Kohut had predicted, the patient's previous intensely negative transference eventually faded as he felt accepted and understood by me.

Kohut felt that the patient had a pathological idealization of his father that was deformed because of the strength and certitude with which the father constantly pointed out his son's shortcomings in a humiliating way. His boss was initially experienced as more powerful and more accepting than the father. He rescued the patient from his feeling of self-hatred and depression when he approved of the patient. With the rejection, by this boss, a profound regression ensued, leading to treatment with me. The patient did not experience me as powerful as the father or as powerful as the overidealized boss. I felt as if I were being experienced as a mother who could accept him, listen to him, as a separate person. Kohut and I kept this discussion going for the length of our consultation.

The patient was very fragile and easily upset, and demanded to be understood. If he was late for an appointment because his train was late or because he had been delayed at work, he would become disorganized, furious at the world for getting in his way and furious at me for not making up the time he had lost. This kind of experience with the patient was very distressing to me; I did not feel that the patient was engaged in analysis as I had been taught to define it. At these times Kohut patiently accepted my frustration, understood how hard it was for me, but emphasized how important it was for me to be there for the patient. The patient needed to feel accepted and engaged in the selfobject transference before the analysis could proceed. It was easier for me to be with the patient after these consultations. However, at times it seemed no matter what I did, I could not soothe his deepest griefs nor relieve his raging flare-ups that resulted from narcissistic injury. It was very frustrating for me to feel as helpless as the patient. Kohut felt the patient was trying to communicate his helplessness and his frustration to me. This response differs from Galatzer-Levy's (this volume) observation that Kohut was not interested in the communication from the patient as picked up by one's countertransference (Racker, 1968), but instead viewed the countertransference response as a limitation of one's ability to treat a patient.

I felt that Kohut really emphasized both points of view. He again pointed out to me that my countertransference anger was getting in the way of understanding what this patient was feeling. At that point, I had lost any capacity for empathy with my patient, and Kohut urged me to try to grasp what my not being available to the patient meant to him. Kohut emphasized that even a psychotic could be successfully analyzed if the analyst could be empathic with the patient. He said that an analyst had to recognize the limits of his ability, rather than blame the patient for being "too sick." I trusted Kohut's experience and knowledge, which helped me when I was with the patient. It seemed as if I were learning how to fly an airplane on instruments without visual cues and had to trust the instrument and teacher at the same time. The situation did encourage me to make more conscious attemps at self-analysis. I attempted to come to terms with my countertransference anger and frustration. Kohut would say, "You were angry with him and, it is dreadfully upsetting to him." He did not want to discuss the countertranference meaning to me unless I was unable to grasp it myself. I suspect he realized that an investigation of my countertransference with him may have led to a more "therapeutic contract," which neither of us had agreed to. Kohut would very astutely ask me, "In what way is this patient correct about you being wrong in your interpretation?" "What element of trust is correct for him given his life experience?" When I made a transference interpretation the patient only felt that I was criticizing him and blaming him for being bad because he was upset.

I can see in retrospect that I used my interpretation of resistance to disavow my own countertransference anger at feeling helpless. Thus, I succeeded in creating a real situation where I was not different from the transference object. A stalemate ensued. Newman (1985) described this well in his paper "Countertransference, Its Role in Facilitating the Use of the Object." Initially I was skeptical about Kohut's approach because it meant changing what I thought of as proper technique, facing my discomfort of the unknown, and facing the helplessness of being with an intensely angry patient who did not seem to change. It was easier to think that this patient was not analyzable than for me to change my clinical stance, which protected me from my discomfort. However, because the supervisory alliance was very positive, it enabled me to stretch myself with a patient whom I could not help with my classical technique. I should acknowledge now with hindsight and more experience that in the initial phase of treatment, neither classical theory nor classical technique was useful in treating this patient. The patient was disorganized because I failed to grasp the transference enactment, which I saw and interpreted as resistance. It was my lack of empathy and understanding due to an improper use of theory that did not apply to this patient at that time. I was confusing psychoanalytic observational data and psychoanalytic theory. Kohut, using his experience-distant theory of the self, helped me be with the patient in an experience-near way. This is probably one of the most difficult concepts that a psychoanalytic student needs to master in his supervised education. Kohut's theory can help one to follow the process and avoid confusing theory with observational data, no matter what the theory is. Younger, less experienced analysts may find self theory as helpful in learning how to follow the patient in an experience-near way. Many experienced traditional analysts can do this, and it is implicit in their technique. They see no need for a new theory.

To return to the case, after about a year of treatment, the patient was still very distraught and often in profound regressions. I had never before worked analytically with this degree of regression in a patient. At these times Kohut suggested, ''The patient doesn't need an interpretation or an explanation but needs to have his feeling accepted by you.'' The patient attempted further contact with the ex-boss who had rejected him and who continued to do so by not acquiescing to this patient's demands and requests for restitution of past wrongs. Kohut's encouragement helped me deal with a pervasive feeling of helplessness and despair that I felt with this patient.

To empathize with how bad the patient felt over disapointment when the reality event seemed untraumatic was difficult for me. It felt that I would be ''gratifying'' the patient and would be establishing an irretractible regressed transference. It was difficult for me to change my way of working. However, persisting in my analytic stance was getting nowhere with this patient. I needed to establish a positive transference to engage the patient. If one does not accept and understand what the patient is saying, how can the patient possibly have an alliance with which to work? Some analysts might say that not interpreting the transference as resistance over a prolonged time would not be analysis because it was gratifying. I simply allowed the selfobject transference to deepen when I no longer interfered with it by interpreting it as resistance. The presence and constancy of seeing an analyst four times per week is also gratifying to a patient. Such gratification cannot be avoided, as it is part of technique, as is understanding the patient and conveying it to him. Basch (1986) points out that Kohut discussed the problem of understanding and gratification:

Empathic understanding implies frustration because the analyst does not meet the overt request made by the patient but only indicates that he understands what the patient is experiencing and, if possible and indicated, interprets the genetics and dynamics of the situation . . . to legitimize a patient's experience by acknowledging that what he is feeling is genuine is not to gratify the wishes being expressed by those feelings . . . frustration is based on the hypothesis that every patient is unconsciously trying to fulfill forbidden, repressed, instinctual wishes, and . . . for the analyst to grant any degree of gratification to the patient is to inadvertently play into resistance by fulfilling rather than analyzing the underlying instinctual demand . . . this is how 'gratification' came to be a dirty word in our field. This overlooks that the greatest gratification a patient can have is to be properly understood. It is the fear of not being understood that makes the patient mobilize wishes for indulgences that are truly not gratifying, i.e., satisfying, and these desires generally fade, once the analyst is able to become empathic with and convey understanding of the patient's unconscious need [pp. 423–424].

Kohut felt that even though this case had a large regressive potential, the patient had enough ego strength for analysis. He did not have many meaningful separate objects, but he had the capacity to relate to people as separate objects with a deep sense of loyalty and fairness if he was not suffering from narcissistic injury. Kohut felt that my analyzing this patient would be limited only by my countertransference response, which constrained my ability to empathize with the patient's experience at the moment. The patient felt at one point that I really did not understand him and that he was getting nowhere with me. He berated me for being inept and unable to help him. The patient was incensed with me and threatened to stop analysis, to prove to the world that I was incompetent. This state gradually faded as the patient began to experience my attempt to understand him.

There was a gradual shifting to a low intensity idealizing transference toward me, and a tentative therapeutic alliance was established. Because of the shift in my attitude, the patient settled down and felt more comfortable over the ensuing months. Kohut had been away for several months on his summer vacation. Upon his return he felt that while he was away the patient had demonstrated that he could "heal" and that I had demonstrated the capacity to accept the patient when he needed to be accepted. However, times of great stress for the patient continued to be fraught with distortions or disavowals of reality. My introduction of reality at those times (a countertransference response) usually caused further disintegration. The patient would again rage at me, wanting me to redress the injury by acknowledging that I had in fact injured him by pointing out reality. The patient knew what he needed.

After about 18 months of treatment the process seemed to be taking hold. The patient found me to be a "usable" object. He could idealize me more comfortably even though I was still not in his "father and ex-boss's league," as he would jokingly and fondly say. It was clear to me clinically that the primary transference to me was as a responsive, understanding, soothing maternal object rather than as the idealized and powerful father figure. He did not regain his cohesion from idealizing me and seeing me as the powerful male figure that he yearned for.

Kohut conceded that he needed me to help him in the reasonable way he desired from his mother. He suggested that the patient needed help in separating from the enmeshment with the father. I felt this could happen only with the establishment of a positive, stable, maternal transference. He could use me as the mother in order to deal with his disappointment and rage toward the father, thereby healing the basic deficit in the mother–child dyad, which he had been unable to do in reality. This was never fully agreed upon by Kohut.

With the establishment of a more stable positive transference, it was suggested that now, in addition to acknowledging the patient's feelings as being valid and important, I needed to explain to him, when he felt that I had failed him, that he was reenacting the past. That is, I had to give him a genetic transference interpretation. This was moving from the stage of understanding to explanation. Now the patient could hear this clearly and not react by feeling blamed. Clearly, establishing a positive relationship by not interfering with the establishment of a selfobject transference was absolutely essential before any interpretation of transference could be made. This process also occurs with a more structured patient, although a well-structured patient does not need as much attention paid to the establishment of an analytic alliance. According to Markson and Thomson (1986) all conflict comes from weakened structure, and the structural deficit is the weakened structure, which leads to structural conflict. Structural deficit means that something is missing in a weakened deformed structure. It is not the absence of structure. The two-stage method of understanding and explanation has applicability to classical cases. Markson and Thomson describe an interesting case of the analysis of oedipal material where they believe ". . . there is no conlict of clinical dimension without underlying deficit" (p. 34).

The case continued with some regressions back to more primitive enactments of anger, generally in response to injuries from my misunderstanding or misinterpreting something the patient was saying or to failures on the part of people in his environment. My own sense of helplessness would be stirred up during these times. Kohut said that the patient was not trying to upset me but was allowing me to experience the sense of helplessness of a deprived, lonely child. Kohut taught me a valuable way of listening to the patient.

I saw Kohut for the last time in July of 1981, when he went away for his summer vacation. The case was going well, and we had made an appointment for the fall upon his return. I received a postcard from him while he was on vacation in Carmel, California, and was very touched that he took the time to write. It was clear that his health was failing. After making a final speech and appearance at a Self Psychology Conference in Berkeley in October of 1981, he returned to Chicago and died four days later. I experienced his death as a very personal loss of both a friend and a teacher. It has been very difficult to separate my personal relation to Kohut, which was warm and meaningful, from my professional experience with him, which was also very important to my professional growth. I think the personal relationship in this supervisory experience was very important to my learning his new theories, which often were contrary to what I had learned in my analytic training. His capacity for empathizing with my struggle with his concepts, and his delight in my learning them, helped immeasurably in the learning process. Being respectfully and empathically treated as a younger colleague was essential to the success of the supervisory process.

I continued with this case for three more years without any further consultation after Kohut's death. The patient terminated the analysis in 1984. He solidified his structural integrity and then began comfortably to experience other people as separate. His relationship with his wife improved, even though there was a selfobject tinge to this marital relationship. There was a markedly increased ability to experience and deal with his spouse as a separate person. He was able to make sacrifices in his own career to further the career of his spouse. During the latter years of the analysis, clearly oedipal material came up in the transference around envy and hostility toward me and sexual feelings toward my wife. These sexual feelings were initially distressing to the patient. He often felt angry and competitive with me, alternating with a positive feeling toward me in both the father and mother transference. There was a working through of these oedipal stage configurations, resulting in a more cohesive self along with stable object relations that were experienced as separate. In classical terms, he had a more mature ego and superego with ''postoedipal'' autonomy over his infantile drives and affects, which had much less intensity as his self structure was strengthened. He was less vulnerable to narcissistic injury and was able to recover quickly. The drives as disintegration products had quieted down as the self healed. He had a greater recognition of my separateness and a greater appreciation and recognition of my feeling states.

The analysis of the selfobject transferences was prerequisite before the oedipal transferences could enter the analysis in an emotional and affective way. Without the analysis of the self-pathology, this patient's oedipal transferences would have been more intellectual, with the affect split off because the self would not have been strong enough to engage them. Had Kohut lived, I think he would have concurred with this, but he would have disagreed about the importance of the analysis of separate object transferences on theoretical grounds.

Further clinical evidence came up having to do with my ongoing difference with Kohut about the nature of the major transference configuration. Quite unsolicited by me (in the termination phase) the patient said that he felt the analysis was very helpful because he experienced me (in the transference) as a "good enough" mother who was there for him, unlike his own mother. This allowed him to get back on track developmentally. There was a slightly idealized father transference in quiet accepting terms, which was different from the constant depreciation of me in the beginning. Once he could experience me as a reliable maternal object he was able to feel good about himself, feeling less vulnerable to injury. As the basic deficit with the mother was healed, he no longer idealized his father as much and saw him more objectively. He no longer was disturbed by the rejection by his ex-boss and renounced him as a significant object. He felt good about himself in a separate, more differentiated way. His capacity to relate to me was on a more separate basis, and the selfobject transferences were more mature. It was also true, in an extratransference way, that this patient was able to deal with his spouse as a separate person. Of course, narcissistic injuries still occurred, but the regressions were shortlived. Through the analysis he was able to internalize my parental function of calming and soothing. He recognized his separateness and identified with my capacity finally to empathize with him. Also in the termination phase it was clear that there was a transference to me both as the father and the mother at an oedipal level. It was the resolution of these higher developmental transferences that enabled this patient to feel separate from me and eventually to experience his spouse as separate without fear of being retraumatized as a selfobject. In addition to mature selfobject transferences, the oedipal transferences were both triadic and separate. The acceptance of oedipal reality did not need to be disavowed with grandiosity or idealization. Kohut did not exclude analysis of oedipal phase transferences, but described them at a selfobject level. The results of this analysis would be acceptable by classical analysts, if these results could be translated into structural terms, that is, oedipal reality testing, mature selfobjects recognized as separate, firm superego, an ego idea, and a more solid ego.

If one deals with the analytic process clinically and is not directed exlusively by one's own experience-distant metapsychology, the usefulness of Kohut's ideas are evident. The metapsychology that Kohut used was different from classical psychoanalysis, although his results were not different in classical terms. Kohut's theory enabled those who used it to do a more complete analysis of preoedipal and oedipal phases than could have been done before. Kohut made an important contribution to psychoanalysis and to those of us whose natural talents were impeded by experience-distant theory that did not allow the natural and normal flowing of empathy that some in our profession employ. To these colleagues this contribution by Kohut is only another set of theories that does not add anything to their clinical stance. Kohut's experience-distant theory of the self allows others to engage their patients clinically in an experience near way. At the same time, there are many who have lost touch with the empathic clinical approach of Freud, and this is a new opportunity for us to regain the past. Merton Gill, at a meeting of the American Psychoanalytic Association in New York in 1979, said publicly from the floor that he did not agree with Kohut's metapsychology, but felt that Kohut had reintroduced empathy, which was being given only lip service by many in psychoanalysis.

These cases and the consultation raise the question of how one defines psychoanalysis and what is analyzability when one clinically is at the cutting edge of this definition with a patient? Metapsychological theory alone does not define psychoanalysis. Psychoanalysis as a techique is based on the development of a transference, its interpretation, and resolution leading to a structural change. A fixed metapsychology based on the transference of impulse and defense is no longer metapsychology; it does not leave room for new theories that can expand and enrich psychoanalysis and allow it to grow as a science. We need a broader definition of psychoanalysis and of transference that will enable us to analyze the patients that classical theory is not as helpful with. Disagreement with Kohut's metapsychology should not cloud one's view of his clinical contributions, which have broadened psychoanalysis for a younger generation of analysts. For others, both in the younger generation and in the older generation, Kohut has created metapsychological problems, which themselves open opportunities to question and define existing theories and clinical positions. My concept of psychoanalysis has unquestionably broadened and deepened as a result of my experience consulting with Kohut.

REFERENCES

Basch, M. (1986), How does analysis cure? An appreciation. *Psychoanal. Inq.*, 6:403–428.

Fleming, J. & Benedek, T. (1966), *Psychoanalytic Supervision*, New York: Grune & Stratton.

Freud, S. (1911), Psychoanalytic notes on an autobiographical account of a case of paranoia. *Standard Edition*, 12:3–82. London: Hogarth Press, 1958.

_____ (1912), Recommendations to physicians practicing psychoanalysis, *Standard Edition*, 12:114–120. London: Hogarth Press, 1958.

_____ (1913), On the beginning of treatment. *Standard Edition*, 12:139–140. London: Hogarth Press, 1958.

Kohut, H. (1984), *How Does Analysis Cure?*, ed. A. Goldberg with P. Stepansky. Chicago: University of Chicago Press.

Markson, E. & Thomson, P. (1986), The relationship between the psychoanalytic concepts of conflict and deficit. In: *Progress in Self Psychology*, Vol. 2, ed. A. Goldberg. New York: Guilford Press, pp. 31–40.

Meyers, S. (reporter) (1981), Panel report: The bipolar self. *J. Amer. Psychoanal. Ass.*, 29:143–159.

Miller, J. (1985), How Kohut actually worked. In: *Progress in Self Psychology*, Vol. 1, ed. A. Goldberg. New York: Guilford Press, pp. 13–30.

Newman, K. (1985), Countertransference—Its role in facilitating the use of the object. Presented to the Chicago Psychoanalytic Society.

Racker, H. (1968), *Transference and Countertransference*. New York: International Universities Press.

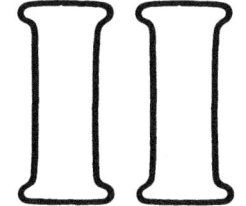

Integration
of Theories

Integrating Self Psychology and Classical Psychoanalysis: An Experience-Near Approach

Robert D. Stolorow

The history of psychoanalysis has been characterized since its early beginnings by the formation of separate and insular schools of thought, divided from one another primarily along metapsychological lines, with little intercommunication or cross-fertilization among the differing viewpoints. A central thesis of this chapter is that psychoanalytic knowledge will be advanced if the clinical understandings obtained from differently situated points of view can be integrated into more encompassing frameworks. To that end, I will consider the formidable problem of integrating the perspectives of psychoanalytic self psychology and classical psychoanalysis. First, I will discuss a number of previous approaches to this problem and indicate why I believe these have not been successful. Second, I will propose two methodological principles through which integration can be approached. And third, I will describe my own attempt, in collaboration with Bernard Brandchaft, to arrive at a more embracing viewpoint through the application of these methodological principles.

Certain preliminary grapplings with the question of integration were already implicit in Kohut's (1971) first book, *The Analysis of the Self*, a work that he later (personal communication) described as an attempt to ''pour new wine into old bottles.'' The new discoveries regarding disorders of the self and selfobject transferences were essentially integrated *into* the Procrustean bed of Freudian metapsychology and

63

voiced in the language of traditional "mental apparatus" psychology and "drive-discharge" theory. Object-instinctual and narcissistic energies were said to follow their own distinct developmental pathways, with each cathecting their respective targets of investment. Fixations along the object-instinctual pathway were thought to result in the formation of classical transference neuroses and a propensity to establish neurotic transferences in the analytic situation, whereas fixations along the narcissistic pathway were seen as resulting in the formation of narcissistic disorders and the corresponding establishment of self-object transferences.

The answer to the question of integration implicit in these formulations was that different theoretical models are necessary for conceptualizing and guiding the treatment of different classes of psychopathology. This approach was made explicit in Gedo and Goldberg's (1973) book, *Models of the Mind*, and in work by Lachmann and me (1976), in which we claimed that a variant of classical theory was appropriate for narcissistic pathology deriving from defenses against intrapsychic conflict, whereas Kohut's ideas were needed for understanding and treating narcissistic pathology rooted in developmental arrests. While this approach to integration was useful in its time, it has since proven to be unsatisfactory. This is because what were formerly conceptualized as distinct classes of psychopathology increasingly came to be recognized as *dimensions of experience* present, with varying degrees of motivational salience, in all persons (Stolorow and Lachmann, 1980, 1981; Stolorow, 1986). Selfobject transference, for example, is no longer viewed as a *type* of transference characteristic of a delimited group of patients, but rather as a *dimension* of all transference that fluctuates in its experiential preeminence throughout the course of analysis (Stolorow and Lachmann, 1984/1985).

Increasingly it became evident to Kohut that the old bottles of classical metapsychology could not contain the new wine of self psychology. Hence, in *The Restoration of the Self*, he (1977) presented self psychology as a new theoretical paradigm, freed from the strictures of Freudian metapsychology and from the doctrine of instinctual determinism. I (1983) have characterized this paradigm as a "developmental phenomenology of the self," because of its central concern with the ontogenesis, structuralization, and psychopathology of self-experience. The explicit formulation of self psychology as a new paradigm made it necessary for Kohut to grapple for a second time with the question of integration, and his proposal at this juncture was that self psychology and traditional Freudian mental apparatus psychology could exist in a complementary relationship with one another. For example, so-called drive conflicts presumably could be viewed *both* from the perspective of classical instinct theory *and* as breakdown products of a fragmenting self. Shane and Shane (1986) have offered a variation on this principle of complementarity in which they suggest that the self-selfobject units of self psychology and the id, ego, and superego structures of classical theory should be assembled into a combined model that can incorporate the advantages of both viewpoints.

Although these formulations of complementary or combined models are not without heuristic value, it is my view that they are theoretically unsound. This is because conceptualizations of self-selfobject experiences and constructions of a drive-discharge apparatus exist on entirely different theoretical planes deriving from completely different universes of discourse. Whereas the former pertain to the experience-near realm of personal meaning, the latter are couched in the assumptions of materialism, determinism, and mechanism that were the heritage of Freud's immersion in 19th-century biology. The two could never truly complement or combine with one another to form the basis for a unified psychoanalytic theory.

Kohut's (1980) third (and, I believe, final) position on this issue was that efforts to integrate self psychology with other theoretical viewpoints, including the classical one, should be postponed until the self-psychological system has become more fully elaborated and consolidated. While this suggestion has much to recommend it from the standpoint of theoretical development within self psychology, it could, if followed as a long-term strategy, result in a form of theoretical parochialism not unlike that which has afflicted orthodox analysis. Periodic articulations between two theoretical perspectives are revitalizing for both.

How, then, might we approach this problem of integrating self psychology and classical psychoanalysis? It is my belief that integration becomes possible by following two basic methodological principles. The first holds that genuine integration can occur only on an *experience-near* plane of discourse, stripped of metapsychological encumbrances. The second maintains that integration takes place through the formulation of new units of analysis that are more *general* and *inclusive* than those of either theory—constructs that can encompass the experience-near understandings acquired from both perspectives.

Let us now apply these two principles of integration to one issue that currently seems to separate sharply the viewpoints of classical psychoanalysis and self psychology—the question of whether inner conflict or selfobject failure should be viewed as primary in the genesis of psychopathology and in the formation of analytic transferences.

Applying the principle of experience-nearness to classical conflict theory, it becomes apparent that when analysts present formulations about drives, if there are any experiential referents for such statements, they consist of *affect states*, such as erotic lust or narcissistic rage (Jones, 1985). Once inner conflict is liberated from the doctrine of instinctual determinism and from the encumbering image of an energy disposal apparatus, and it is recognized that the conflicts with which classical analysis has always been concerned pertain not to drives but to affect states, then the theoretical chasm that has separated conflict psychology and self psychology begins to close (Stolorow, 1985). When it is further recognized that not only does affect lie at the heart of the phenomenology of inner conflict, but that the *integration* of affect is central to the structuralization of the self, then a pathway for synthesizing the two theoretical viewpoints begins to open up before us.

Daphne Socarides and I (1984/1985) have proposed that selfobject functions pertain fundamentally to the integration of affect into the organization of self-experience, and that the need for selfobject ties pertains most centrally to the need for attuned responsiveness to affect states in all stages of the life cycle. From this standpoint, the two categories of selfobject need initially delineated by Kohut (1971, 1977) point to the critical role of mirroring responses in the integration of affect states involving pride and expansiveness, and of soothing responses from idealized sources of strength in the integration of affect states involving anxiety and helpless vulnerability. Foreshadowing a bridge between conflict theory and self psychology, Socarides and I wrote:

> Affects can be seen as organizers of self-experience throughout development, if met with the requisite affirming, accepting, differentiating, synthesizing, and containing responses from caregivers. An absence of steady, attuned responsiveness to the child's affect states creates minute but significant derailments of optimal affect integration and leads to a propensity to dissociate or disavow affective reactions because they threaten the precarious structuralizations that have been achieved. The child, in other words, becomes vulnerable to *self-fragmentation* because his affect states have not been met with the requisite responsiveness from the caregiving surround and thus cannot become integrated into the organization of his self-experience. Defenses against affect then become necessary to preserve the integrity of a brittle self-structure [p. 106].

Brandchaft and I (Stolorow and Brandchaft, 1987) explicitly extended these formulations to a reconceptualization of conflict formation:

> The specific intersubjective contexts in which conflict takes form are those in which central affect states of the child cannot be integrated because they fail to evoke the requisite, attuned responsiveness from the caregiv-

ing surround. Such unintegrated affect states become the source of lifelong inner conflict, because they are experienced as threats both to the person's established psychological organization and to the maintenance of vitally needed ties. Thus affect-dissociating defensive operations are called into play, which reappear in the analytic situation in the form of resistance. A defensive self-ideal is often established, which represents the self purified of the "offending" affect states that were perceived as intolerable to the early surround, and the inability to fully embody this affectively purified ideal then becomes a continual source of shame and self-loathing. It is in the defensive walling off of central affect states, rooted in early derailments of affect integration, that the origins of what has traditionally been called the *dynamic unconscious* can be found [p. 246].

We formulated two broad classes of affect states that regularly become sources of structuralized conflict in the context of faulty affect attunement: those that accompany the child's developmental strivings (e.g., feelings of pride, expansiveness, efficacy, rebelliousness, competitiveness, and emergent sexuality) and those that are reactive to threats, injuries, or disruptions (e.g., anxiety, sadness, disappointment, shame, guilt, and rage). This conceptualization of conflict formation, we further contended, holds critical implications for the analytic approach to resistance:

When defenses against affect arise in treatment, they must be understood as being rooted in the patient's expectation or fear *in the transference* that his emerging feeling states will meet with the same faulty responsiveness that they received from the original caregivers. Furthermore, these resistances against affect cannot be interpreted as resulting solely from intrapsychic processes within the patient. Such resistances are most often evoked by events occurring within the intersubjective dialogue of the analytic situation that for the patient signal a lack of receptivity on the analyst's part to the patient's emerging feeling states, and therefore, herald a traumatic recurrence of early selfobject failure. . . . Thus, although the persistence of resistance reflects the continuing influence of preestablished organizing principles (the repetitive aspect of the transference), the resolution of resistance and the establishment of new modes of experiencing require careful analytic attention to the specific intersubjective contexts in which the defensive reactions arise and recede [pp. 246-247].

What emerges from the foregoing formulations of selfobject functions, conflict, and resistance is, in very broad brushstrokes, a *bipolar conception of transference* (see also Ornstein, 1974). At one pole of the transference is the patient's need for the analyst to serve as a source of requisite selfobject functions that had been missing or insufficient during the formative years. In this dimension of the transference, the patient hopes and searches for a new selfobject experience that will enable him to resume and complete an arrested developmental process. At the other pole are the patient's expectations and fears of a transference repetition of the original experiences of selfobject failure. It is this second dimension of the transference that becomes the source of conflict and resistance.

I believe that a well-conducted psychoanalysis is characterized by inevitable, continual shifts in the figure-ground relationships between these two poles of the transference, as they oscillate between the experiential foreground and background of the treatment. These oscillations correspond to shifts in the patient's psychological organization and motivational priorities that occur in response to alterations in the tie to the analyst—shifts and alterations that are profoundly influenced by whether or not the analyst's interpretive activity is experienced by the patient as being attuned to his affective states and needs. For example, when the analyst is experienced as unattuned, foreshadowing a traumatic repetition of early selfobject failure, this invariably brings the conflictual and resistive dimension of the transference into the foreground, while the patient's selfobject needs are, of necessity, driven into hiding. On the other hand, when the analyst is able to analyze accurately the patient's experience of selfobject failure, demonstrating his attunement to the patient's reactive affect states and thereby mending the ruptured tie, the selfobject pole of the transference becomes restored and strengthened and the conflictual/resistive/repetitive dimension tends to recede into the background.[1] The analyst's empathic comprehension of these shifting figure-ground relationships between the two poles of the transference should determine the content and timing of transference interpretations (Stolorow and Lachmann, 1984/1985). Furthermore, I believe that the mode of therapeutic action of the analysis will differ, depending on whether it is the selfobject or conflictual dimension of the transference that occupies the position of foreground at any particular juncture of the treatment (Stolorow, in press).

CONCLUSION

It has been my aim to demonstrate that both our theoretical construc-

---

[1]At certain other times, the patient's experience of the analyst's attunement may actually *heighten* the conflictual and resistive aspect of the transference because it stirs the patient's walled off selfobject longings and archaic hopes, along with his dread of the retraumatization that he fears will follow from the exposure of these longings and hopes to the analyst. I am grateful to Drs. Evan Brahm and Anna Ornstein for reminding me of this point.

tions and our clinical understandings greatly benefit from our remaining within the domain of the experience-near. From a firmly planted stance within this domain, it is clear that psychic conflict and selfobject failure should not be seen as dichotomous, but as dimensions of experience that are indissolubly interrelated. A focus on affect integration and its derailments illuminates the intersubjective contexts of selfobject failure in which inner conflict takes form. The concept of an *intersubjective field* (Atwood and Stolorow, 1984; Stolorow, Brandchaft, and Atwood, 1987) established between the psychological worlds of child and caregiver, or of patient and analyst, provides a unit of analysis that is broader and more inclusive than either intrapsychic conflict or the self-selfobject relationship. By encompassing both the conflictual and selfobject dimensions of experience, as well as their mutual interplay and oscillating figure-ground relationships, the concept of an intersubjective system offers a promising, experience-near pathway for synthesizing the clinical understandings of classical psychoanalysis and self psychology into a unified psychoanalytic framework.

REFERENCES

Atwood, G. & Stolorow, R. (1984), *Structures of Subjectivity*. Hillsdale, NJ: Analytic Press.

Gedo, J. & Goldberg, A. (1973), *Models of the Mind*. Chicago: University of Chicago Press.

Jones, J. (1985), The concept of drive. Unpublished manuscript.

Kohut, H. (1971), *The Analysis of the Self*. New York: International Universities Press.

———— (1977), *The Restoration of the Self*. New York: International Universities Press.

———— (1980), Reflections on *Advances in Self Psychology*. In: *Advances in Self Psychology*, ed. A. Goldberg. New York: International Universities Press, pp. 473–554.

Lachmann, F. & Stolorow, R. (1976), Idealization and grandiosity: Developmental considerations and treatment implications. *Psychoanal. Quart.*, 45:565–587.

Ornstein, A. (1974), The dread to repeat and the new beginning. *The Annual of Psychoanalysis*, 2:231–248. New York: International Universities Press.

Shane, M. & Shane, E. (1986), Self change and development in the analysis of an adolescent patient: The use of a combined model with a developmental orientation and approach. In: *Progress in Self Psychology*, Vol. 2, ed. A. Goldberg. New York: Guilford Press, pp. 142–160.

Socarides, D. & Stolorow, R. (1984/1985), Affects and selfobjects. *The Annual of Psychoanalysis*, 12/13:105–119. New York: International Universities Press.

Stolorow, R. (1983), Self psychology—A structural psychology. In: *Reflections on Self Psychology*, ed. J. Lichtenberg & S. Kaplan. Hillsdale, NJ: Analytic Press, pp. 287–296.

———— (1985), Toward a pure psychology of inner conflict. In: *Progress in Self Psychology*, Vol. 1, ed. A. Goldberg. New York: Guilford Press, pp. 193–201.

———— (1986), On experiencing an object: A multidimensional perspective. In: *Progress in Self Psychology*, Vol. 2, ed. A. Goldberg. New York: Guilford Press, pp. 273–279.

———— (in press). Transference and the therapeutic process. *Psychoanal. Rev.*

———— Brandchaft, B., Atwood, G. (1987), Developmental failure and psychic conflict. *Psychoanal. Psychol.* 4:241–253.

_____ _____ Atwood, G. (1987), *Psychoanalytic Treatment: An Intersubjective Approach*. Hillsdale, NJ: The Analytic Press.

_____ Lachmann, F. (1980), *Psychoanalysis of Developmental Arrests: Theory and Treatment*. New York: International Universities Press.

_____ _____ (1981), Two psychoanalyses or one? *Psychoanal. Rev.*, 68:307–319.

_____ _____ (1984/1985), Transference: The future of an illusion. *The Annual of Psychoanalysis*, 12/13:19–37. New York: International Universities Press.

Chapter 4

Pathways to Integration: Adding to the Self Psychology Model

Morton Shane
Estelle Shane

Our topic for this chapter is "Pathways to Integration," but it could as well be "Pathways Back to Integration," for in a sense integration is not new to self psychology at all. Its beginnings were in unity with classical analysis, a creative extension of the mainstream. And when Kohut, in *The Restoration of the Self* (1977), set self psychology on its new and independent course, the linkage to classical analysis was still maintained through the concept of complementarity. Over the subsequent years, and through the publication of his last posthumous book, even as Kohut more and more conceptualized self psychology as standing free of traditional analysis, he nevertheless maintained a connection to the mainstream. To our knowledge, he never dismissed the idea that basic training in analysis requires classical understanding of neurotic conflicts, defenses, and the dynamic unconscious. In extending psychoanalysis, he could not, and did not, break his ties with crucial and basic psychoanalytic knowledge. This is not to ignore the fact that Kohut's agenda was at first to cloak his new ideas in familiar terms in order to make them seem less foreign and more acceptable to the psychoanalytic establishment, and only later, and then somewhat gradually, to free self psychology from many outmoded psychoanalytic concepts. In this process, the self-in-the-narrow-sense and complementarity fell by the wayside. We believe that with this jettisoning effort vital aspects of mental functioning, essential to psychoanalysis,

71

were either discarded or left unacknowledged. But, if self psychology is truly to assume, and then maintain, a leadership role in psychoanalysis—in effect to *become* the mainstream—it must find a way to address a broadened field of normality and pathology. Many concepts inherent in the tripartite model, and still necessary to the field, must be included under the expanded umbrella of self-psychological theory.

This is a good time for self psychology. The psychoanalytic need for a concept of a superordinate self is increasingly acknowledged (e.g. Meissner, 1986); but if the self is to be effectively superordinate, it must carry with it the idea of an entity that functions all of a piece, at the same time that it functions with inner conflict, tension, and disparity. Kohut's vision of the self encompasses both, but with too little emphasis on the latter; the modern tripartite model of mainstream analysis encompasses both, with too little emphasis on the former. We do not believe it constitutes too great a strain on the theoretical capacity of psychoanalysis to conceptualize a self that can do both *equally*, that is, function at times in a holistic fashion and at times in conflict within itself. In effect, we are saying that a selective integration is necessary and can best be accomplished through a sanitized and updated tripartite addition to the self psychology model. We did not always conceptualize integration in this way, so before going further with this proposal, we would like to review briefly what we have learned from some of our past efforts, which can be thought of most accurately as ''difficulties in the pathway toward integration.''

It has been nearly ten years since we (Shane and Shane, 1980) first attempted to integrate psychoanalytic models of self development. At that time, we viewed the psychoanalytic self from objective, subjective, and reconstructive vantage points, with the main thrust being to highlight the concurrences in developmental perspective among Kohut (1971, 1977), Mahler, Pine, and Bergman (1975), and Piaget and Inhelder (1969). Kohut (1980) responded to this effort with a significant elaboration of his conception of normal development, clarifying his divergences from mainstream analysis in two important ways: one, that the mainstream goal of striving toward autonomy masks a moralistic stance that self psychology, with its emphasis on the necessity for selfobject experiences throughout life, assiduously avoids; and, two, that the mainstream view of aggression as innately destructive does not fit with data derived from the clinical situation. Kohut's point was that concurrence between his views and the mainstream could never be accomplished because of these divergences. In subsequent papers, we have responded to Kohut's criticisms of our first effort in ways designed to bring to the mainstream insights from self psychology such as these, and to demonstrate their compatibility. Thus, to our view,

Kohut was correct: the classical concept of innate destructiveness is not only unnecessary as a postulate, misleading in the clinical situation, but it is also inconsistent with developmental studies on infants and children, as noted, for example, in the observational research of Parens (1979) who is, after all, a classical analyst in the Mahler tradition.

In terms of the other point Kohut took issue with, autonomy from objects versus lifelong dependency on selfobjects, again Kohut was right in pointing to a hidden moralistic stance, but to our minds what is hidden in that stance is the gender bias so prevalent in our culture: that a real man is independent of others; that it is feminine, and therefore reprehensible, to find in oneself a need for a supportive surround. Kohut's valuable insight that the need of the self for self-sustaining selfobject experience is lifelong, on the other hand, should be balanced by the reminder that as development proceeds and the individual progresses from infantile to mature selfobject needs, the reduction of reliance on infantile-archaic selfobjects is a sign of greater maturity and stability of the self. Transmuting internalization, the result of optimal frustration, gratification, and responsiveness in selfobject experience, does lead to meliorative developmental structural change in the self (see Greenberg and Mitchell, 1983, p. 369). It follows, then, that the reliance on selfobjects will thereby be altered and even diminished, though the ability to turn to selfobjects when necessary, and to establish such ties, is a sign of maturity and health. The alteration of self-cohesiveness, self-firmness, and self-harmony that results from transmuting internalization requires more specific investigation.

We believe such efforts would demonstrate the establishment of an equilibrium between autonomy from and dependence on selfobject ties in the healthy, mature self, representing a necessary addition to the selfobject theory of motivation. As a corollary, the capacity to be available to serve selfobject needs of another must be factored in as a measure of maturity; this capability is obviously essential for adequate parenting and other mature relationships, including being a psychoanalyst or therapist. To repeat, we do not believe that development toward autonomy need be antithetical to self psychology, nor need it, when balanced by the selfobject concept, carry with it a moral stance.

In summary, Kohut dismissed the idea of integration in this first attempt. The reasons he gave were enlightening but did not discourage us from further efforts. In a more recent paper (Shane and Shane, 1986), we attempted to combine the bipolar self with the tripartite model of the psyche. To facilitate the integration of these models, modifications were required in each, as follows: the bipolar self is equated with the psyche as a whole, as the tripartite model has always been so equated. The tripartite model is firmly removed from any direct connection to biology, enabling one to see id, not as Freud had conceptualized it, but instead in line with the modern conceptualization of impulse as affective and emotional striving, or psychological wish. This permits us to view the tripartite model as exclusively within the realm of the psychological, just as self psychology is conceptualized within this realm. The superego is freed of energic conceptions of innate destructiveness turned on self. In combination, each of these models is enriched and enhanced, with the analyst being provided a larger, more tightly woven net to explain the work with clinical phenomena; both neurotic and self-pathological aspects of the patient can be addressed, understood, and interpreted. Again, we want to respond to one criticism of this approach; (e.g. Meissner, 1986) that is, the contention that there is an inherent incompatibility between these two models because they exist on different levels of abstraction, the self model being considered experience-near, and the tripartite, experience-distant. We argue that distinctions between phenomena on these grounds are, at best, extremely difficult to make and agree upon. Observations in the clinical situation cannot be made with any coherence without an informing theory, which inevitably establishes a distance from the "raw data." In this sense, all theories are experience-distant; and to determine from the data which one is more distant is not feasible, and it is conceptually possible to reintroduce into the theory of self psychology concepts drawn from the tripartite model.

As we indicated, self psychology began as integrated with classical analysis and for some years continued to freely utilize classical concepts. For example, in *The Analysis of the Self*, Kohut (1971) nicely depicted vertical and horizontal splits to account for defensive actions within the psyche, such as disavowal and repression. Representations of objects as well as selfobjects were acknowledged, as was the distinction between the object and the selfobject concepts. Energic considerations were specific, carrying with them, unfortunately, all the inconsistencies that energic concepts have always carried in psychoanalysis. While since that time self psychology wisely dropped energic concepts, it also, less wisely we believe, either dropped or played down defenses; representations, or schemata; the object concept as contrasted with the selfobject concept; and a persistent focus on the dynamics of the dynamic unconscious. Of course, at no time in the history of self psychology has the dynamic unconscious been ignored, but a dynamic unconscious requires the concept of dangerous and unacceptable mental contents that must be defended against. This means that phenomena that in mainstream analysis are termed ego and superego dynamic-defensive functions must be accounted for in self-psychology. Such a dynamic view of defense is in addition to self-psychological postulates regarding defensive and compensatory structures.

Specifically, we think we must once again allow for the inclusion of an object concept in general in addition to a selfobject concept. It is not sufficient to say that selfobject relationships are primary and central in disorders of the self, whereas difficulties in ordinary object relationships are secondary and not pathogenic; after all, self psychology addresses issues beyond self-disorders, including normal development, normal oedipal phase conflicts other than the Oedipus complex per se, and pathological states other than those found in self pathology. For example, Basch (1986), along with Greenberg and Mitchell (1983), contends, and we agree, that the mother must serve as more than just a selfobject. There is a theoretical need, then, for a means to represent functions and interactions between self and true object, as well as self and selfobject. For a parent to be in mature empathic contact with his or her child, the child must be experienced as an object, not as a selfobject. This we have called the capacity for otherhood (Shane, 1988). The child needs to be seen as having its own center of initiative and its own unique program of development. The same is true for analysts and therapists vis-à-vis their patients. When instead, the child or patient is experienced as a selfobject, the parent or analyst is serving his or her own self-interest rather than the child's or the patient's. If this is a correct statement, then we need an object concept to deal with it.

To turn to another point, self psychology employs as a primary motivational system the seeking for selfobject experiences to shore up weaknesses in the self. In the interest of distancing the theory from a drive motivational system, forbidden or dangerous desire is ignored on two grounds: one, desire is seen as an expression of a biological drive; and, two, desire is not conceptualized as primarily pathogenic, save when it is postulated as breakdown product. However, if the oedipal phase, normal or even joyous as it may sometimes be, is to be considered "oedipal" in any sense of the word, both parents must be conceptualized as sensuously and sexually desired, with this desire being experienced by the child as forbidden, that is, disapproved of, to some degree, by parental figures. Pathogenic or not, theoretical capacity must be present to handle such phenomena. Our assertion is that self psychology, to be a more comprehensive theory, needs some kind of tripartitelike theoretical system to be adapted to or amalgamated with the bipolar self.

In relation to the process of interpretation in the psychoanalytic situation, a dispassionate view of Kohut's contribution will reveal a difference in accent, rather than a difference in substance, vis-à-vis the traditional mode. Kohut says that explanation, or interpretation, is optimally frustrating to the patient and leads to the formation of psychic structure. While he acknowledges that insight is useful, he views it as less centrally important than the total experience of being understood and helped to understand. Classical analysis, on the other hand, yields a central place to insight, but many classical analysts stress, in addition, the crucial role of structural change necessary for any insight to be effective (e.g. Schlessinger and Robbins, 1983). The psychoanalytic concept of working through attests to this. In an earlier paper, one of us (Shane, 1979) noted that the well-observed time lapse between insight and psychic change could be understood in terms of developmental process in the patient in response to the analytic situation. Such an understanding of this lapse is over and above the necessary attainment of multiple insights that emerge over the course of an analysis (Greenson, 1967; Brenner, 1987). Kohut strengthens our conviction that some vital and permanent changes take place within the self, enabling the insight to hold and to make a difference in the patient's total functioning. This is to say that interpretations leading to insight are imparted by the analyst, who, at the same time, is having a developmental impact on his patient. A significant effect on this developmental impact is the experience of being understood, but we must leave room for all developmental influences the analyst has on his patient, including such supportive measures as are conceptualized in a developmental orientation.

For example, self psychology focuses on the analytic ambiance, as do developmentalists who also refer to the analytic ambiance as the therapeutic or working alliance (see Shane, 1979). The latter has fallen into disfavor in classical analysis and has never been much acknowledged by self psychology. We see it as a helpful addition to self psychology to give a place to the therapeutic alliance in the analytic situation, in order to elucidate structural changes that make analysis more possible as the selfobject transferences progress developmentally. An improved therapeutic alliance enables a patient to tolerate both empathic disruptions and hitherto warded off mental contents and so deepens analytic experience and therapeutic effects. While in classical analysis (e.g., Brenner, 1982) one who is not capable of an adequate working alliance is simply not analyzable, rendering the working alliance an unnecessary construct, self psychology widens the scope of analyzability, providing a therapeutic/working alliance with a developmental dimension, namely, the self-selfobject relationship. This is especially the case in the alter ego selfobject transference, wherein the skills and talents required for analysis can be supported.

Finally, we believe self psychology should introduce a modern view of the superego into the pole of ideals and standards, a superego purged of outdated concepts of innate destructive aggression turned on the self as well as the obligatory link to oedipal conflict resolution. There is clinical value in adding such a superegolike concept to the bipolar self; it would provide conceptual space to distinguish between two types of internalization frequently viewed in the transference. That is, the self-psychological concept of transmuting internalization can be described as a seamless addition to self-structure; a selfobject function is internalized without an object tag. This may be distinguished from superego functions that do have a dynamically unconscious object tag. In our view, both kinds of internalization are demonstrable clinically. For example, a patient prides himself on unswerving honesty. In the course of analysis, this ideal is discovered to be emotionally linked to love for his mother, who herself revered honesty. This same patient also requires, for smooth functioning, self-orderliness, but this standard is not linked to a definitive object. Rather, it appears to be a selfobject function acquired through transmuting internalization. Both qualities, honesty and orderliness, seem equally stable and mature. However, while though a breach of honesty carries with it a threat of loss of object love and the experience of guilt, a failure in orderliness is responded to with only mild shame and a dysphoric feeling of disorganization. We do not believe that identification can always be conceptualized as an archaic form of transmuting internalization; therefore, self psychology needs to account for mature identifications, most clearly discerned in the pole of ideals and standards (but in other sectors of the self as well).

To end aphoristically, by adding Guilty Man to Tragic Man we come to a closer approximation of reality, namely, Protean Man.

REFERENCES

Basch, M. F. (1986) How does analysis cure?, An appreciation. *Psychoanal. Inq.*: 6:403–428.
Brenner, C. (1982), *The Mind in Conflict*. New York: International Universities Press.
_____ (1987), Working through: 1914–1984, *Psychoanal. Quart.*, 56:88-108.
Greenberg, J. R. & Mitchell, S. A. (1983), *Object Relations in Psychoanalytic Theory*. Cambridge, MA: Harvard University Press.
Greenson, R. R. (1967), *The Technique and Practice of Psychoanalysis*, Vol. I. New York: International Universities Press.
Kohut, H. (1971), *The Analysis of the Self*. New York: International Universities Press.
_____ (1977), *The Restoration of the Self*. New York: International Universities Press.
_____ (1980), Summarizing reflections. In: *Advances in Self Psychology*, ed. A. Goldberg. New York: International Universities Press, pp. 473–554.
Mahler, M. S., Pine, F. & Bergman, A. (1975). *The Psychological Birth of the Human Infant*. New York: Basic Books.
Meissner, W. (1986), Can psychoanalysis find its self?, *J. Amer. Psychoanal. Assn.*
Parens, H. (1979), *Aggression in Childhood*. New York: Aronson.
Piaget, J. & Inhelder, B. (1969), *The Psychology of the Child*. New York: Basic Books.
Schlesinger, N. & Robbins, F. P. (1983), *A Developmental View of the Psychoanalytic Process*. New York: International Universities Press.

Shane, M. (1979), the developmental approach to working through. *Int. J. Psychoanal.*, 60:375–382.

———— (1988), The struggle for otherhood: Its significance in adult development. Presented at the Southern California Psychoanalytic Society, Los Angeles, CA, February.

———— Shane, E. (1980), Psychoanalytic Developmental Theories of the Self: An integration. In: *Advances in Self Psychology*, ed. A. Goldberg. New York: International Universities Press, pp. 23–46.

———— ———— (1986), The bipolar-tripartite Self: An integration. In: *Progress in Self Psychology Vol. 2*, ed. A. Goldberg. New York: Guilford Press.

Chapter 5

Reflections on Integration of Theories

KOHUT'S VIEWS ON INTEGRATION
Jule P. Miller, Jr.

Morton and Estelle Shane and Stolorow outline two differing but valuable approaches to the integration of self psychology and classical psychoanalysis.

The Shanes' approach is similar to that of Kohut: they would integrate the two views by combining, in various ways, parts of the self psychology and classical models. As Lachmann mentioned earlier, this is a mixed-models approach. Stolorow rejects this approach on the grounds that the conceptualizations involved in the two systems are incompatible. He then develops a different and promising approach to integration aimed, in part, at avoiding conceptual incompatibility.

But are the arguments compelling? And must we therefore abandon the mixed-model approach? I think not, especially if we are willing to tolerate a degree of conceptual difficulty as our work proceeds—a departure from ideal theoretical fit that often accompanies creative work—for example, the work of Kohut and the work of Freud.

Stolorow's objections are illustrative of other, comparable positions in the literature. Stolorow states:

Although these formulations of complementary or combined models are not without heuristic value, it is my view that they are theoretically unsound. This is because conceptualizations of self-selfobject experiences and constructions of a drive-discharge apparatus exist on entirely different theoretical planes deriving from completely different universes of discourse. Whereas the former pertain to the experience-near realm of personal meaning, the latter are couched in the assumptions of materialism, determinism, and mechanism that were the heritage of Freud's immersion in 19th century biology. The two could never truly complement or combine with one another [this volume, p. 65].

I believe this argument is flawed in that it depends on an imprecise paring of the levels being considered. Stolorow compares experience-near aspects of self-psychological theory to experience-distant aspects of traditional theory, and of course they do not match. What can be compared are the more experience-distant concepts of self psychology with the more experience-distant concepts of traditional analysis. For example, the concept of the bipolar self, which Stolorow himself, quite rightly, considers to be experience-distant, metapsychological, and of doubtful utility, should be paired with the more experience-distant formulations of the structural theory, including the view of the mind as a drive-discharge apparatus. These experience-distant conceptualizations would be on roughly the same level. On the experience-near level, conceptualizations involving empathically perceived self-selfobject experiences would be correlated with conceptualizations involving empathically perceived impulse-defense configurations or wish-avoidance configurations. The referent of each of these sets of concepts is empathic immersion in the experience of the patient, and they are roughly conceptually compatible.

Therefore, an integration based on mixtures or combinations of the two models is, in principle, tenable and is one important way in which resolution of the problem should be sought; other approaches, such as the elegant one of Stolorow and his colleagues, should proceed concurrently.

My principal objection to each of the contributions of Stolorow and the Shanes is their insufficient appreciation, in my opinion, of the very substantial work of integration that was done by Kohut, work that remains the most important on this subject to date. Kohut's consideration of issues of integration was continued by him in *How Does Analysis Cure?* (1984), which can be viewed as an extended consideration of the relationship between, and the integration of, self psychology and more traditional views.

Kohut's considerations of integration in *The Analysis of the Self* (1971) and *The Restoration of the Self* (1977) are well known. His published remarks at conferences continued to express his concerns with integration. For example, at the Boston Conference in 1980 (see Lichtenberg and Kaplan, 1983) Kohut said, "First of all, and this argument needs no elaboration, self psychology adds something to traditional analysis; it does not substitute for it. It can, therefore, hardly be argued that self psychology is impoverishing analysis by supplementing the traditional point of view with the vista obtained from a new vantage point" (p. 400). In this same discussion, he further states, "My answer is that I am much more of a drive psychologist than some of the critics of self psychology. Self psychology does not replace drive psychology anymore than quantum physics replaces the physics of Newton. We are dealing with different vantage points, shifts in outlook, complementarity of perspective" (p. 397).

In the final phases of his thinking on the relationship of self psychology to classical analysis, Kohut's reliance on complementarity declined, as noted by the Shanes. It was largely replaced by emphasis on two other concepts: the concepts of an intermediate sequence of impulse-defense material, and the concept of disintegration products, appearing after a fragmentation of the self and containing intensified and disordered drive elements and regressive defenses against them.

This shift derived from the fact that as self psychology developed Kohut no longer viewed it primarily as an alternative explanation for clinical phenomena of equivalent importance. Rather, he increasingly saw self psychology as the central, fundamental position of analytic psychology and believed that it subsumed the classical position. It did not eliminate the classical position, certainly not entirely, but contained it and treated classical concepts and findings, in essence, as "special cases" within self psychology. This is analogous to viewing Newton's laws of motion as useful special cases within the more valid, larger viewpoint of modern physics. For example, as posited by self psychology, a pathological Oedipus complex is seen as a frequently occurring, special-case deterioration of the normal oedipal stage.

Let me illustrate with a brief clinical instance. When I first began studying with Kohut late in 1978, I presented clinical material from an analysis. In one session the patient began with a dream, clearly an oedipal dream, with prominent negative oedipal, unconscious homosexual elements. The patient's associations went from there to dream references to castration fear, then to anal issues, and then to oral preoccupation. This entire sequence followed my canceling a session with a patient. Kohut's comment on the material was that it was a most interesting intermediate sequence of "classical" material. By this he meant that this sequence of oedipal to anal to oral had coherence and validity, and could be understood meaningfully in traditional terms and interpreted in its own right. He added, however, that he would understand the significance of this intermediate sequence very differently as a self psychologist from the way he would have understood it from the viewpoint of classical analysis years ago.

The trigger for the sequence was, of course, my cancelation of the analytic session, producing a rupture in the self-selfobject bond. This led to fragmentation of the patients's self and to intensification of impulse-defense configurations as a result of that fragmentation. In other words, disintegration products were formed as a consequence of the fragmentation. These intensified impulses and primitive defenses led to the intermediate sequence that has been described. Theoretically, the most basic aspect of the sequence was a rupture in the selfobject bond that initiated it and the restoration of the bond through my empathic comprehension of the situation and its interpretation. Kohut considered the interruption and subsequent restoration of the self-selfobject bond as anchoring, fore and aft, the intermediate sequence.

While such an intermediate sequence is theoretically of secondary importance, it may at times be of great clinical significance. The intensified and distorted drive and defense elements may be involved in the formation of classical neurotic systems through well-known channels, including compromise formation. More important, the intensified impulse-defense elements may be involved in the deterioration of normal, developmental oral, anal and oedipal stages into the corresponding pathological complexes.

For a clinical illustration from Kohut himself, I wish to quote an important passage from *How Does Analysis Cure?* (1984). Kohut states,

> For a long time during the analysis of an oedipal transference, for example—that is , for a long time during the analysis of an Oedipus complex that has been remobilized in the transference—the analyst will properly function as the analysand's selfobject only if he focuses his interpretations on the latter's incestuous desires and death wishes and on the well-known conflicts of ambivalence that accompany these drive-fed impulses. Should the analyst attempt to bypass the Oedipus complex and push the patient prematurely toward the failures of the oedipal selfobjects of childhood which led to the Oedipus complex, the analysand will feel misunderstood and retreat whether by an open resistance and protest or, one of the strongest resistances encountered, by external compliance [p. 67].

In this important statement, Kohut affirms that the root cause of oedipal pathology is self-pathology. However, in clinical work, when oedipal pathology is in the foreground of the therapeutic scene, it must be dealt with on its own terms, and dealt with in this way until the underlying self pathology begins to come into focus. This means that for prolonged periods in some treatments the focus may be on oedipal material narrowly conceived, even in the best conducted self-psychologically informed psychoanalyses. This, in my opinion, is a deeply meaningful integrative position.

Kohut's description of normal stages of development and pathological complexes is both a major advance over traditional theory, and, at the same time, broadly integrative. Kohut states that he believes there are normal phases of development that include and subsume the classical Freudian positions such as the oral, the anal, and the oedipal. He believes that under conditions of adequate parenting, these phases, while involving conflict and suffering, are normal stages of growth and their outcome is increased maturation. A pathological condition, for example the pathological Oedipus complex, occurs when the parenting in the oedipal phase has been inadequate, leading to a fragmentation of the self and to pathological intensification of oedipal impulses and reactive castration fear. Kohut is explicit in the *Restoration of the Self* (1977) that "the normal oedipal phase, considered as a growth phase, involves sexual feelings towards the mother on the part of the boy, competitive and rivalrous feelings towards the father and resultants fears of bodily mutilation" (p. 230). However, Kohut maintains that these feelings normally remain within levels of intensity that permit the oedipal experience to be, in net balance, a positive growth phase. If, however, the child is met in the oedipal stage with pathological parenting of a type that Kohut describes in detail, this may lead to a fragmentation of the self, to a resultant pathological intensification of oedipal feelings, so that the boy's sexual attraction to his mother becomes crudely sexual and his competition with his father violently aggressive, leading to an intensification of retaliatory castration fears and the development of an abnormal and pathogenic Oedipus complex.

Kohut's beautiful conception enables us to work with oedipal material and to do it full justice, from a clearly defined self-psychological position. Kohut's views answer the problems of the pathological Oedipus complex more satisfactorily than they are answered by traditional analysis. It explains all the phenomena that the traditional view explains. In addition, it provides us with a reasonable explanation for how a pathological Oedipus complex comes about—for its cause—an explanation that is largely lacking in traditional analysis.

Kohut's self psychology can explain all the pathological material of traditional analysis, and a great deal more besides. It does this by subsuming the more experience-near concepts of traditional analysis within the encompassing conception of the psychology of the self in the larger sense. Much of traditional psychopathology is then seen as based on a "special case" deficit in and distortion of normal development, mediated in part by mechanisms such as the formation of disintegration products and of pathological intermediate sequences. The bedrock of all psychopathology remains, of course, inadequate formation or disruption of self-selfobject bonds.

I believe that a good deal of the mixed model integrative work outlined by the Shanes was already done by Kohut. However, much additional work in this direction remains. I agree with the Shanes, for example, that more understanding of the place and role of superego functions within the psychology of the self is needed. I hope their valuable work will proceed and will include a renewed emphasis on their developmental perspectives.

Stolorow's direction is broadening, promising, and in many places conceptually clarifying. I know that he and his colleagues are working to extend, add specifics, and flesh out their model. I would be interested in hearing, for example, how he would approach some of the classical clinical issues—such as the pathological Oedipus complex and neurotic symptom formation, from his point of view.

These contributions are a valuable part of the exciting, ongoing efforts to integrate self psychology with classical analysis. All of us who address this challenge face together the ancient problem of valuing and retaining the best that we have, while building on it and altering it in creative and meaningful ways.

REFERENCES

Kohut, H. (1971), *The Analysis of the Self.* New York: International Universities Press.
_____ (1977), *The Restoration of the Self.* New York: International Universities Press.
_____ (1984), *How Does Analysis Cure?* New York: International Universities Press.
Lichtenberg, J. & Kaplan, S., eds. (1983), *Reflections on Self Psychology.* Hillsdale, NJ: The Analytic Press.

COMMENTS ON "COMPLEMENTARITY" AND THE CONCEPT OF A COMBINED MODEL
Robert J. Leider

There are many areas of agreement among the Shanes, Stolorow, and myself. Foremost, we agree that an overall *model* of mental functioning, capable of organizing the concepts and observations central to self psychology, integrating the phenomena central to classical psychoanalysis, and illuminating clinical practice, is desirable. Such a model optimally should also be consistent with knowledge about psychological development and function obtained from nonpsychoanalytic methodologies.

The Shanes and Stolorow each propose a model they assert to be suitable for these purposes. But while they share the same goal, the models they propose are very different and, to my mind, not compatible with each other.

Turning to the Shanes' contribution, I would first emphasize several additional areas in which I am in agreement with the authors. The reformulation of "drive" as an aspect of an affective configuration, and the recognition that aggression is not primarily destructive, are congruent with my views. Furthermore, I support their assertion that self psychology has given too little attention to the functions of, and interaction between, the object and the self.

However, perhaps the point most central to the Shanes' position is their view that "many concepts inherent in the tripartite model and still necessary to the field must be included under the expanded umbrella of self psychology theory . . . it must carry with it the idea of an entity that functions all of a piece, at the same time that it functions with inner conflict, tension, and disparity." And that "a selective integration . . . can best be accomplished through a sanitized and updated tripartite addition to the self psychology model" (p. 72).[1]

Here my views differ. The clinical observations and phenomena described from the perspective of classical theory must be encompassed by a more inclusive model, but I do not believe that the essential concepts of the tripartite model, or a sanitized version, can be retained, nor that a suitable model can be constructed by the superimposition of one upon the other. (Kohut, 1977, pp. 242–243, was of a similar opinion.)

The tripartite model was designed to organize observations regarding impulses, dangers, conflict, prohibition, and guilt. Its *central concept of motivation* is the "drive." Normal psychological development and psychopathological phenomena are organized around and viewed from the perspective of the "drive" and its vicissitudes, satisfaction, taming, or frustration, in relation to an object. This narrow focus has restricted the utility of the tripartite model, leading to attempts to broaden its explanatory power by various emendations, e.g., Anna Freud (1965), Hartmann (1964), Kohut (1966), and Jacobson (1964), to name just a few. None of these approaches has been satisfactory; all have been correctly criticized on theoretical grounds and the unsuitability of the tripartite model for a task it was not designed to perform has been repeatedly demonstrated.

---

[1]P. Ornstein, and others, have observed that such a "sanitized and updated" tripartite model would probably not be acceptable to classical drive theorists as a suitable starting point for an integrated model.

The model of the *superordinate self* is designed from a different frame of reference, for a different purpose: that of explicating the gradually increasing cohesion, strength, and harmony of the self, the role and function of the selfobject in this process, and various pathological states that occur when this process is derailed. In this model, *the central motivational factors stem from the needs or poles of the self for a responsive selfobject matrix*. Drives are accorded a minor position in psychological development and pathology: "The primary psychological configurations in the child's experiential world *are not drives*" (Kohut, 1977, p. 171).

For these reasons, I conclude that the two models are not compatible and can not be integrated in the manner suggested by the Shanes, not because of different levels of abstraction (Meissner, 1986; Stolorow, this volume), but because they make fundamentally different assumptions regarding the central motivational factors in development and pathology.[2]

Stolorow's contribution is a severely condensed series of interlocking conceptions and arguments explicated in greater detail, force, and elegance in a number of books and papers written by himself and in collaboration with Atwood, Brandschaft, Lachmann, and D. Socarides, which must be consulted to understand his views.

Stolorow is embarked on a reconsideration of psychoanalytic observations, formulations, and models, with the aim of correcting various errors, offering a series of reformulations, and suggesting a new system, the *intersubjective field* as "a promising, experience-near pathway for synthesizing the clinical understandings of classical psychoanalysis and self psychology into a unified psychoanalytic framework" (p. 69).

Several assumptions, with which I am in agreement, underly this enterprise: that the empathic, introspective mode of observation defines the empirical and theoretical domain of psychoanalysis; that the mechanistic, deterministic assumptions of drive metapsychology be rejected; and that it is desirable to integrate understandings derived from different points of view. I am also in agreement with many of the clinical observations and formulations offered by Stolorow, but I do not understand the need for, nor superiority of, the new system, the intersubjective field, over some of the models discarded by Stolorow as wanting.

Stolorow asserts that this system resolves the issue whether inner conflict or selfobject failure should be viewed as primary; permits a closing of the chasm that separates conflict psychology and self psychology; and better allows for the conceptualization of, and the clini-

---

[2]Greenberg and Mitchell (1983) reach the same concusion.

cal approach to, shifting aspects, or dimensions, of the transference.

His argument regarding conflict, with which I agree, is that drive concepts are better formulated as affect states, and that conflict results from a derailment of affect integration consequent to a failure to evoke the requisite attuned responsiveness from the caretaking surround. An understanding of the development of conflict in childhood, and of its emergence in the clinical situation, is provided by this formulation. It does open a "pathway to integration," *by explaining conflict from a self-psychological perspective.*

Stolorow considers Kohut's (1977) concept of complementarity, and the hierarchical model of Gedo and Goldberg (1973), and rejects these models as pathways to integration for several reasons. First, he believes that the shifting conflictual and selfobject dimensions of the transference are not adequately represented by these formulations. Additionally, he would reject the former because of retention of remnants of a mechanistic drive-discharge conflict apparatus, far from subjective experience; and the latter because "what were formerly conceptualized as two distinct classes of psychopathology came to be recognized as dimensions of experience present" (p. 64). Finally, Stolorow proposes the *intersubjective field* as a more satisfactory organizing theory.

In my view, however, the arguments for the rejection of these models are not persuasive. Stolorow's description of complementarity and its theoretical faults is apt only to the concept as *first described* by Kohut (1977, pp. xv, 77), when he was still struggling with the scientific and political ramifications of the shift in paradigm which he ultimately fully explicated.

Slightly later he was clear and definite that the self in relation to selfobjects is central and basic to all classes of psychpathology: "I will not hide my belief that in the long run a psychology of the self will prove to be . . . indispensable even with regard to the areas where the psychology of drives and defenses now does the job" (p. 98). And

> . . . it is not a libidinal drive that, psychologically speaking, attains its momentum in the child . . . the drive experience is subordinated to the child's experience of the relation between the self and the selfobjects. . . . It changes our evaluation of the significance of the libido theory on all levels of psychological development in childhood [and] . . . it changes our evaluation of some forms of psychopathology which classical theory viewed as being caused by . . . fixation on or regression to this or that stage of instinct development [p. 80].

With the latter view, Kohut rejected the original meaning of complementarity. But the concept was retained, purged of the faults

Stolorow described, in Kohut's description of the analyses of oedipal neuroses and fluctuating levels of transference:

> The analytic process will, therefore, not only deal with the oedipal conflicts per se but also, in a subsequent phase or, more frequently, more or less simultaneously (though even then with gradually increasing emphasis), focus on the underlying depression and the recognition of the failures of the child's oedipal selfobjects [1984, p. 5].

and in other comments elsewhere (1977, pp. 228, 229; 1984, p. 22); descriptions that I find similar, though not congruent, with Stolorow's concept of the bipolar structure of the transference, imbricated in his model of the intersubjective field.

In conclusion, I am in agreement with Stolorow's propositions concerning the elimination of the remnants of mechanistic drive theory, his reformulation of drive and conflict, his thoughts on transmuting internalization, and his thoughts on the curative process. But I disagree with his rejection of a hierarchical model that includes complementarity, and with his assertion of greater power for the model of the intersubjective field.

REFERENCES

Freud, A. (1965), *Normality and Pathology in Childhood*. New York: International Universities Press.

Gedo, J. E. & Goldberg, A. (1973), *Models of the Mind*. Chicago: University of Chicago Press.

Greenberg, J. R. & Mitchell, S. A. (1983), *Object Relations in Psychoanalytic Theory*. Cambridge, MA: Harvard University Press.

Hartmann, H. (1964), *Essays on Ego Psychology*. New York: International Universities Press.

Jacobson, E. (1964), *The Self and the Object World*. New York: International Universities Press.

Kohut, H. (1966), Forms and transformations of narcissism. *J. Amer. Psychanal. Assn.*, 14:243–272.

_____ (1977), *The Restoration of the Self*. New York: International Universities Press.

_____ (1984), *How Does Analysis Cure?* Chicago: University of Chicago Press.

Meissner, W. W. (1986), Can psychoanalysis find its self? *J. Amer. Psychoanal. Assn.*, 34:379–400.

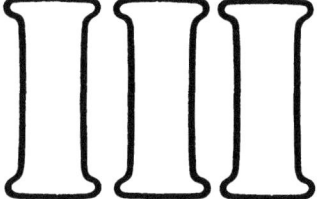

Development

Chapter 6

Constitution in Infancy: Implications for Early Development and Psychoanalysis

Barbara Fajardo

Infant development research has in recent years intrigued psychoanalysts, stimulating new ideas and confronting old assumptions about a "tabula rasa" newborn who is molded by experience and environment. There is now a large body of evidence from developmental studies that support the view of the newborn as a uniquely organized, active participant in its own experience, and even having significant influence in determining the nature of his environment and caretaker responses to him (Scarr and McCartney, 1983). This paper summarizes some preliminary findings of an ongoing research project suggesting that even in the earliest observable preterm development, individual infants make their own unique constitutional contribution to their development and their experience of the environment.

Until very recently, with the books by Lichtenberg (1983) and by Stern (1985), the neonatal period was usually ignored or dismissed by psychoanalysts as prepsychological. Mahler, Pine and Bergman (1975) call this age, to two months postterm, the "autistic period" and bypass it to begin their discussion of development with the "symbiotic period." They characterize the autistic period by an absence of cathexis and responsiveness to external stimuli. Spitz (1965) is more generous about acknowledging the capacity of the full-term newborn to organize responses to the environment, but he attributes this ability to universally shared, innate, reflexlike behaviors grounded in biological maturation, with no contributions from learning. Departing from this tradition, Stern (1985) has marshaled evidence from many studies of infant development, proposing that the period in human life from full-term birth to two months is important in the development of the sense of self. He uses the term "emergent self" to describe the process and product of becoming organized, which is the sense of self that forms during this period.

> Infants begin to experience a sense of an emergent self from birth. They are predesigned to be aware of self-organizing processes. They never experience a period of total self/other undifferentiation. There is no confusion between self and other in the beginning or at any other point during infancy. They are also predesigned to be selectively responsive to external social events and never experience an autistic-like phase [p. 10]

Stern believes that this sense of self, like the other three successively developed senses of self (core self, subjective self, and verbal self), remains a process that continues to function actively throughout life. The early sense of self is not replaced by later ones, but rather it continues to grow and coexist (p. 11) with the later forms.

While Stern places the onset of the emergent self at term birth, its onset could perhaps more precisely be defined as the beginning of the fetus' capacity to learn and to experience. From 32 weeks postconception, or six to eight weeks before term birth, most researchers agree (see Parmalee and Stern, 1972) that infants begin to have increasing capacities for alert and attentive states, for awareness of environment and for their own experiences of dysphoria and comfort, and for learning in interaction with the environment. These capacities enable infants even at this early age to begin experiencing themselves as having a locus of intentionality with causal impact on the environment and caretaker. Inasmuch as psychoanalysis has always pursued the origins of experience in its genetic theory, this earliest origin of the experience of self will be intriguing to self psychologists. The conception of the self as an independent center of initiative is shared by many infant psychologists and researchers, who see infants as active, aware participants in their experience.

The objectives of the study described here are: (1) to observe the development of the earliest capacities for self-organization, (2) to explore the contributions of environment and caretaking to these emerging capacities, and (3) to note some consequences of the vicissitudes in these earliest self-organization capacities for later development. The term "self-organization" here is an index to the sense of self. Our data about the infants' capacities for self-organization are the observable patterns of their state organization. There are four major classes of state:

quiet sleep, active sleep, drowse, and alert. As infants develop an increased capacity for self-organization, their states become more clearly differentiated, and each state begins to be more regularly accompanied by clusters of particular behaviors. For instance, sucking becomes rhythmic and occurs particularly during quiet sleep and not in other states. With development, this flow of activity becomes less disruptable by environmental stimuli or physiological sensation. In other words, behaviors and responses gradually become more regulated or defined by an overarching state. Infants who are more capable of this self-organization appear to feel more comfortable and secure and have fewer dysphoric or painful moments. State organization is evaluated using the data obtained by an observer who sits quietly by the infant's bassinet for two to four hours between feedings and for every 30-second period records state, behaviors, and physiological events.

Ninety-five or more percent of the time between feedings, infants usually are in sleep states or in some transition phase between them. Summarily defined, quiet sleep appears more peaceful and often more physiologically organized to the observer than active sleep. *Quiet sleep*, by term age, can be accompanied by rhythmic sucking, regular respiration, low muscle tone, rhythmic startles, no major body movements, and closed eyes. In contrast, *active sleep* gradually becomes associated with patterns of rapid eye movements; closed eyes; frequent body, limb or facial movements; high muscle tone; and irregular respiration. *Drowse* is a waking state, a transition between sleep and alert, which is usually brief and may not ever occur at all. The awake state is characterized by open eyes, eye movements with some visual fixation, or some apparent attentiveness to stimuli of environmental or internal physiological origin.

The research objectives grew out of a background of clinical experience with premature infants. We first met them in the Special Care Nursery and continued to follow them as patients in a Pediatric Developmental Clinic. It is frequently the case that low birthweight premies after nursery discharge are difficult for their mothers in ways that are independent of their medical problems. For instance, an unusually high number of premies have sleep disorders, such as not sleeping through the night until the second year. Many babies and young children are noticed to have idiosyncratic aversions, vulnerabilities, or sensitivities to certain sensations or disruptions, for example, to loud noises and tightly fitting clothes. And a higher number than in a normal population will not tolerate a wide range of responses from mother and seem more particular about how they need her to behave with them. These characteristics can be understood as deficits in a capacity for self-organization or self-regulation. Similar characteristics have been observed and documented by other researchers (see Field, 1982). Probably an important contributing factor to the sensitivities of these babies is the inadvertently chaotic and disrupting nursery environment where they must spend the first couple of months of life, with special life support systems. Although these conditions may be mandated by medical needs, from a psychological perspective, events in the environment are intense, unpredictable, unpatterned, and unrelated to the infant's attempts to self-regulate.

Nonetheless, many infants in our low birthweight premature group develop normal or typical state regulation capacities in spite of prolonged and early exposure to the chaotic and disruptive nursery. If so many infants suffer psychologically and even medically in the nursery environment, one wonders how some other infants (equivalent in their medical condition) still manage to develop normal self-organization capacities. This points to the possibility of still a third factor underlying the development of self-organization, that of innate or constitutional influences, in addition to factors related to the trauma of prematurity and the influence of early nursery environment.

To begin teasing apart the influences of these three factors on emerging self-organization, we instituted an alternative environment in one part of the nursery that is designed to be unchaotic, quieter, and with reduced activity, dimmer lights, demand feeding, and respect for day/night cycles. We have chosen healthy, growing premies for our subjects and have assigned half of them to the intervention environment and half to the regular nursery environment. We observe our subjects twice for state organization, once at 32 weeks, just before they are placed in one of the two environments, and again at 36 weeks, which is the end of the intervention phase and just before their discharge to home. After discharge, we evaluate them clinically and developmentally at several points throughout their first three years of life. Our oldest infants now are about a year old.

We are finding that environment is an important influence on the development of self-organization. All infants placed in the developmentally sensitive environment we provided progressed in the expectable normal direction, some improving dramatically over the four weeks of their exposure to this condition, whereas most infants in the regular nursery environment worsened or made no developmental progress.

The altered nursery environment produced infants who had more of the developmentally expectable improvements in quiet sleep, including more time spent in quiet sleep with longer episodes, and an increased organization within quiet sleep (that is, absence of movements and presence of rhythmic sucking). The infants in the regular nursery progressed less and even worsened: the percentage of quiet sleep *decreased* rather than increased as it should. Infants in the altered nursery were also superior to the ones placed in the regular environment in their developmental progress with active sleep organization, particularly manifested in the duration of REM episodes within this state. The infants remaining in the regular nursery continued to show more startle/tremor behavior and more undirected body movement than those in the altered nursery.

While it would not be surprising to anyone that environmental conditions influence development, it is perhaps unexpected that so little is required of an intervention to be helpful to these infants. Basically, the intervention can be characterized as the reduction of disruption and overstimulation and the introduction of features of predictability (patterns and cycles) and contingencies related to the infants' states. Nothing really has to be "done to" the infants; to develop spontaneously, they need only to be left alone in a supportive background. When infants are not exposed to this phase-appropriate and supportive environment, as is the case in the regular nursery environment, many deteriorate or manifest a developmental delay.

As mentioned earlier, however, not all infants in the regular environment deteriorate; one out of four improve in spite of the odds. While chaos and overstimulation are clearly harmful in varying degrees to the emerging self-organization capacities, there are some infants who seem more resilient and develop normally in spite of the pathogenic influences of the nursery. This suggests that the extent of needs for the phase-appropriate environmental background is variable among infants. Some infants appear to be more vulnerable and less resilient than others, a vulnerability that seems biologically based, because for these tiny, premature infants it cannot be related to earlier, fault-producing psychological experience with an environment.

To illustrate the range of individual variations in constitutional resilience and vulnerabilities, two very different infants will be described. Both were in the intervention nursery environment. Each weighed about two pounds at birth and has had a smooth medical course. Throughout the first year of life, both babies manifested discernable continuities in behavior and probably in their experience of the world. From their birth age of 28 weeks postconception, their mothers were free of apparently serious pathology and were involved with and attentive to them.

Darla was a highly organized infant at 32 weeks postconception (eight weeks preterm). During our three-hour observation, she cycled through her states with smooth, brief transitions, and all her states were steadier and more prolonged than would be expected for her age.

She easily established rhythmic behaviors such as sucking and rapid eye movement patterns, and her startles during a lengthy quiet sleep period were also rhythmic. We have noticed that infants who are more capable of establishing these rhythms tend to be calm and not easily disruptable, and Darla was a good example of an infant who had a remarkable capacity for self-soothing. Even at this young age, she was able to accomplish successful and frequent hand-to-mouth movements. Particularly notable were her lengthy awake states, as she lay calmly and intently surveying her surroundings. She was apparently able to experience a cause-effect relationship between her eye movements and her sensations from vision. This seemed to be a pleasurable experience, one she prolonged and repeated on other occasions.

Five months later, at six months of age, or three months postterm, she was a quiet and visually attentive infant who especially enjoyed the visual-perceptual part of the developmental assessment that involved being shown a variety of interesting visual patterns. While mother and baby were comfortable and easy together, Darla did not particularly like to be held and cuddled and preferred visual to tactile and kinesthetic stimuli. Mother reported that Darla enjoyed sitting in her infant seat watching things at home and did not like to be jostled or roughly played with. This information was congruent with a continuity wherein Darla became more organized and experienced more well-being or security when she initiated visual activity and exploration of something she experienced as interesting and somewhat novel. Visual perceptual experiences were an important self-soothing behavior for her. Mother recognized this about Darla, respected it, and encouraged her in visual explorations while avoiding overstimulating her with tactile and kinesthetic interactions.

Tracy was very different from Darla. At 32 weeks, Tracy was almost constantly tremorous or startling. Quiet sleep and active sleep were not differentiated, and most of the time she was in a poorly organized active sleep state. The brief periods of quiet sleep were marked by large body movements and thrashing movements. Tracy was also very reactive to noise from the environment and to stimuli originating from her internal physiological processes. She was not observed to have any awake states.

As an older infant, at six months of age (or what would be three months if she had been full-term), Tracy was a quiet baby with many smiles but few vocalizations. Mother was quiet with her, did not urge or demand her to respond in a dialogue, and mostly was engaged in caretaking and soothing. Her manner seemed appropriate and sensitive to the kind of baby Tracy was. She remarked that Tracy was sometimes very sensitive and irritated by things. For instance, she had a strong aversion to tightly fitting hats, and she did not like to be held a lot. During the evaluation of visual responsiveness, she was alert and attentive and absorbed by the stimuli, but she did not explore and scan so much as she was riveted by the stimuli. Although she was responsive and attentive to the sights presented, she did not initiate visual perceptual experiences in the way we noticed was an outstanding feature of Darla's behavior.

We saw Tracy again at ten months chronological age, or seven months postterm. At this time, she was a sober baby, watchful, and without the vocalizations expected for her age. She was hypertonic and reactive to abrupt, unfamiliar stimuli, for instance, startling at the sound of a door slamming and crying when she heard another baby's cry in the next room. She was unusually attached to mother, feeling safe only when touching her. When shown an interesting new toy, she attended with intense interest but without the joy and exploration that most babies express at her age. Tracy appeared to be using her mother's protecting and soothing functions as compensation for the self-soothing and self-regulating she was not able to do on her own.

Tracy has a constitutional vulnerability to being painfully over-whelmed, disorganized, and unregulated, which is continuous with her behavior earlier. She has always had few resources to calm herself and to maintain steady states without interruptions. More than most babies, she needs her mother to soothe and smooth things out for her, which could put the mother-child relationship under strain, although at this time the mother was doing an excellent job in responding to her baby's needs.

We propose that there is a group of more vulnerable infants, like Tracy, who improve less dramatically in the calmed-down nursery and who deteriorate even more severely in the regular environment. Maybe these infants have a greater need for the provision of active soothing and organizing functions from the environment, such as an oscillating mattress, because of a vulnerability in their inner resources to self-organize. Perhaps this more pronounced need for a particular environmental responsiveness in certain of our premies is germane to the concept of the selfobject. The average infant manifests an emerging self, a phase-appropriate center of initiative; in contrast, the vulnerable child, with the self in danger, is the infant in need of the caretaker's selfobject function. The vulnerable infant is unable to spontaneously maintain a phase-appropriate cohesive self. In other words, the experience of a selfobject is not essential to stimulate or propel the normal development of early infancy for the average or well-endowed child, in the average or better environment. But it is particularly relevant to the experience of infants who are either constitutionally vulnerable to disorganization or fragmentation or are placed in danger of disorganization by an unempathic environment. If we think of emotional development as occurring *spontaneously* in the average child in the average environment, then the experienced need for a selfobject function emerges only when there is a specific disorganizing influence from within the child or from the environment and caretakers. The inability of the child to recover developmental momentum or equilibrium from this point could lead to a developmental deficit.

Some component of a person's need for a soothing or organizing selfobject function to reorganize after a disruption may be related to constitutional factors. In this regard, it is striking that among the first eight babies studied, who now are around a year old, there is one who is a failure-to-thrive child. As a newborn, she was in the regular nursery environment and deteriorated more than any other child in that group over the four weeks between nursery evaluations. This unusual deterioration suggests that this infant was more constitutionally vulnerable than most to self-disorganization or fragmentation and probably requires more empathy from the caretaker and environment than an average child. She exemplifies a child in need of more experiences of the selfobject in order to develop normally. As the diagnosis of failure-to-thrive implies, this child did not have an empathically capable mother who could provide the needed selfobject functions. Although this is the only case of failure-to-thrive in our study so far, early nursery observations of this child's poor self-organization capabilities lead us to propose that there has been a mismatch between child and mother that is related to a vulnerability of the child as well as to an incapacity in mother. This child was probably more difficult to comprehend empathically than the average infant and clearly needed more from the nursery environment to support normal development. Nursery observations of this infant indicate that this vulnerability can be observed early on in poor capacity for self-organization.

It may be that certain children more than others will not easily experience environmental and maternal responses to them as empathic. This dimension of difference among infants and children cannot be explained as a matter of organic central nervous system damage, although sometimes constitution and organic deficits may overlap and aggravate each other. To what extent do children create the experience of the unempathic parent? Raising this question helps to maintain the proper intrapsychic focus on the experience of the child rather than interpersonal interactions in questions concerning parental failures in empathy. Genetic reconstructions of empathic failures in psychoanalysis are reconstructions of the child's experience and not of what actually took place in an interpersonal context. Another, less constitutionally vulnerable child might have reacted quite differently to the same parental responses.

In our early follow-up phase, we are finding certain continuities between the infants' self-organizing capacities in the nursery and their needs for empathic mothering responses later at one year of age. Infants capable of organized states in the nursery are not as disrupted by insensitive maternal behavior after discharge. Conversely, infants who manifest more early disorganization tend to require more maternal regulation and sensitivity. While we cannot be certain for our six- to twelve-month olds how much the need for particular regulating maternal responses has grown out of the interactive history between infant and mother, it does seem that some part originates with constitutional factors first observed in the nursery.

We are seeing many instances in follow-up of subtle continuities in self-organizational capacities and styles of self-soothing. We are also seeing how the mothers' responses and caretaking styles are appropriately influenced by their often accurate perceptions of these characteristics in their infants. It does not seem that the differences among our developing children can be sufficiently accounted for by variations in the empathic capacities of their mothers.

When we consider implications for treatment situations with adults or older children, these preliminary factors and speculations from our study raise a question about how much a patient's deficit in self-soothing and self-regulating is originally constitutional and how much is evolved out of the interactive history with parental figures. This question is not meant to diminish the importance in technique of a dynamic focus. Indeed, it is sometimes necessary to have a prolonged period of working with and observing a patient from a psychoanalytic view of transference phenomena before the therapist can be certain about constitutional factors. However, the possibility of constitutional factors may explain some limitations in what can be accomplished in a particular treatment situation, for instance, with chronically and pervasively anxious or overwhelmed patients. Some developmental deficits, understood as constitutional rather than dynamically based, could indicate certain educative parameters in treatment. For instance, a patient may have to accept that he has vulnerabilities to certain experiences that lead to disruptions of self-esteem. He could learn in treatment specific strategies for protecting himself and avoiding stimuli that lead to the danger of fragmentation, without requiring that those vulnerabilities be resolved by analysis. Indeed, in some cases such vulnerabilities *cannot* be resolved in analysis or psychotherapy. These constitutional vulnerabilities or strengths can be understood as an aspect of analyzability, not as defining particular diagnostic categories. We encounter nuances of these characteristics in every kind of patient we see.

Self psychology has expanded the objectives of psychoanalytic treatment beyond the neuroses and has stimulated exciting and useful treatment alternatives in our work with many patients. Even so, we must be mindful of the limitations of theory and of our experiences with more intractable disorders in patients who, like certain of our newborns so vulnerable to pathogenic environments, are never really free of their need for the safety and regulating function of a treatment relationship and who do not develop a robust self-regulatory capacity even with the most careful analysis. At the other extreme, we must remember those patients who have dismal histories and unempathic environments throughout development, who nevertheless are highly responsive to treatment and surprise us in their ability to make use of the analysis or psychotherapy. These patients are perhaps like our more resilient infants, who continue to develop their self-regulatory capacities even in the unempathic and chaotic nursery environment. As we learn from these clinical phenomena and from observing the development of infants, we can reflect on the dynamic concepts of self and selfobject as having important constitutional underpinnings. Perhaps future research will further specify constitutional influences on the need for selfobject experiences and on the capacities to have that kind of experience and to experience empathy from another person.

REFERENCES

Field, T. (1982), Affective displays of high-risk infants during early interactions. In: *Emotion and Early Interaction*, ed. T. Field & A. Fogel. Hillsdale, NJ: Lawrence Erlbaum Associates.

Lichtenberg, J. D. (1983), *Psychoanalysis and Infant research*. Hillsdale, NJ: Lawrence Erlbaum Associates.

Mahler, M., Pine, F. & Bergman, A. (1975), *The Psychological Birth of the Human Infant*. New York: Basic Books.

Parmalee, A. & Stern, E. (1972),Development of states in infants. In: *Sleep and the Maturing Nervous System*, ed. C. D. Clemente, D. P. Purpura & F. E. Mayer. New York: Academic Press.

Scarr, S. & McCartney, K. (1983), How people make their own environments: A theory of genotype environment effects. *Child Development*, 54, 424–435.

Spitz, R. (1965), *The First Year of Life: A Psychoanalytic Study of Normal and Deviant Development of Object Relations*. New York: International Universities Press.

Stern, D. N. (1985), *The Interpersonal World of the Infant*. New York: Basic Books.

Chapter 7

Reflections on Development

THE SELFOBJECT EXPERIENCE
OF THE NEWBORN
Michael F. Basch

Dr. Fajardo has given us a clear, interesting, and deceptively simple statement about the early state of the self. I say it is deceptively simple because, for me at least, it calls attention to the need to reexamine the meanings that we attach to our basic vocabulary—not just words like selfobject and empathy, but words like psychology and self. Therefore, in a roundabout way, I will here try to answer the question that Dr. Shane raised in the first part of her discussion, namely, Can we think of selfobject experiences as already occurring at the beginning of life? Can what accounts for the variability in the adaptation of the prematurely born infants be considered something psychological? Many would say no, and might add that any extrapolation from infant behavior, or at least from early infant behavior to later stages of development is not warranted. I disagree with that negative position because, for me, what is psychological is a phylogenetic or evolutionary question and not one of individual development. To put it another way, it is not the nature of behavior, but how it is generated and directed, that decides for me whether or not to call the outcomes of this or that brain function "psychological."

All life, at any level, is a dynamic enterprise. This means that it depends on information processing; that is, stimuli from the environment must be registered, interpreted, and then responded to in an appropriate manner. In animals below the mammalian level, the evoked response to meaningful signals is *instinctually* determined; that is, once released, an inherited, specific program for action runs its course. Biologists use the word drive, or instinctual drive, to indicate that in mammals the bond between stimulus and response is not so tightly coupled and that within limits the brain, the organ responsible for processing information leading to behavior, permits some variation in action programs to take place by allowing for modification of old, as well as a development of new feedback and feedforward cycles. Simply put, mammals can learn; they can adapt their behavioral strategies to changing constraints imposed by the environment.

I will call psychological whatever takes place at the interface between the environment and a brain capable of modification. In other words, I reject the division of life into the biological and the psychological, and say instead that psychology is an aspect of biology, referring, as I said, to the study of those events that take place at the brain/environment interface and dispose toward behavior.

When behavior is not totally predetermined by inherited instinctual programs for survival, once the possibility of choice exists, an animal must have some sense of functioning as an individual entity separate from its surroundings. This need is met by a new system that develops at the interface of brain and surround. It consists initially of inherited programs for perceptual transformations. These perceptual capacities are then modified and extended by the feedback and feedforward cycles that are established by the choices made in the interaction with the environment. The information-processing mediating structure that translates the instinctually inherited blueprint for the preservation of the individual and of the species into behavior that is geared to carry out those aims is what I call the self, or, preferably, the self-system. In this way, psychology becomes the study of the self-system and encompasses human behavior at every stage of life, whether prenatal or postnatal. For this reason I cannot accept Kohut's (1977) suggestion that, early on, the self exists only in the mother's perception as a virtual self. Similarly, though I am very much in favor of Stern's (1985) book, to which Dr. Fajardo referred, I also do not much like the term "emergent self," for the self and its functions are already in evidence during the first two months of life.

Dr. Fajardo's work and that of other infant researchers lets us see the earliest attempts of the self to manage the disorganization created when the organism is subject to overstimulation. The prematurely born infant is a most instructive experiment in nature that can teach us something about empathy and the selfobject experience and the difference between the two.

Empathy, the capacity to find one's way into the subjective experience of another, is shown by removing infants from the overstimulating and inappropriate environment of the average nursery and placing them in one that takes into account and eliminates the harsh, arrhythmical, distressing cacophony of light and sound that is the lot of the average premature baby in the hospital. Did Dr. Fajardo, empathic with the premature infant's state, provide these lucky babies with a selfobject experience? Not necessarily. As she points out, there are infants who are able to thrive even in the unempathic surroundings of the average premature nursery. The self-system is not endangered in such an infant but, rather, is functioning competently as the center for the generation and organization of information. (Notice that I did not say that the self is functioning as a center for independent initiative [Kohut, 1977] for we are always part of transactions with others, past or present. The competent self is capable of initiating action, but independence of initiative is, accurately speaking, an illusion.) As Kohut (1971) originally formulated, it is the absolutely or relatively endangered self that is in need of selfobject experiences. Here, of course, empathic understanding assists in providing that needed selfobject input. The relatively endangered self would be the one that is overstimulated by the tumult of the nursery but, once removed to healthier surroundings, is able to take over the ordering process once more in a phase appropriate way. The absolutely endangered self is found in those premature babies who even in optimal surroundings clearly signal by their distress and dysphoria that their self organization cannot mediate between the brain's need for order and an otherwise *not* excessively stimulating environment.

As Dr. Fajardo makes clear, differentiating between the patient who as an infant was subject to an unempathic environment and the infant whose constitutionally endangered self leads him to experience his parental environment as unempathic is at best an uncertain business. What we see are patterns of tension management or mismanagement that are either carried forward and contaminate later stages of development, or else are awakened at a later date interrupting what looks like reasonable developmental progress, probably indicating that there was trauma in that early phase. Trauma that, though sealed over, was not healed by later compensatory structure formation.

A large number of our patients present us with an example of what happens when early damage in tension management, rather than being neutralized by cognitive maturation, infiltrates it and renders it relatively useless. This is the basis of so-called borderline pathology, whatever symptomatic form it may take. Prolonged empathic immersion, which Kohut so often spoke about, is required if the capacity for the formation of a narcissistic selfobject transference is to be fostered in these individuals. It is this development that will then allow for transmuting internalization and the formation of a competent self system. What, operationally speaking, is it that we actually do to prepare the ground for this to happen? Basically, our intervention can be characterized as reducing disruption and overstimulation, and introducing features of predictability and contingencies related to the patient's state. These words are, of course, lifted directly from Dr. Fajardo's description of the nursery environment she devised, and are as applicable to the treatment of these adult patients as to the treatment of the premature babies that Dr. Fajardo described. What matters is not the age of the patient, but the patterns that we see unfold before us, whether in the cradle, in the chair, or on the couch.

I, for one, will be eager to hear more from Dr. Fajardo as her research progresses and gives us further insight into the formation of the self system.

REFERENCES

Kohut, H. (1971), *The Analysis of the Self*. New York: International Universities Press.
_____ (1977), *The Restoration of the Self*. New York: International Universities Press.
Stern, D. N. (1985), *The Interpersonal World of the Infant*. New York: Basic Books.

THE CLINICAL VALUE OF CONSIDERING
CONSTITUTIONAL FACTORS
Estelle Shane

Dr. Fajardo's paper concerns the observed infant objectively perceived by the researcher in an experimental situation. This view can be contrasted to the reconstructed infant, intersubjectively perceived by the analyst in the clinical situation. We all know that the two situations are not congruent, that a leap of faith and scientific inference are required to make the one contribute to the other. Yet, of necessity, we all make this leap to enable us to deepen our clinical experience. The here and now of the therapeutic situation is always informed by the clinician's sense of normal and pathological development in general and by what in that development is most germane to the therapeutic moment.

Fajardo cogently illustrates this point. Her effort provides data that permit a more accurate view of infancy and its implications for later development in the hope that our reconstructions in analysis might come that much closer to the mark. Examining the interpersonal events of infancy, she provides strong evidence of a link between constitutional predisposition and the capacity for self-organization. Her research illustrates the technique that Stern (1985) has described, that is, discovering the means for allowing infants to answer questions researchers want answered. The question Fajardo wanted answered was, How can infants tell us of their capacity for self organization, of their own sense of self? She discovered the infant could answer that question by revealing the capacity to regulate internal states. Correlations could then be made between this early capacity for state regulation and the later capacity for self regulation.

Fajardo asked the further question, What variables make a difference in development? Is it just the quality of the facilitating environment and the extent of trauma that may combine to either augment or to inhibit self development, or might there be a third variable, constitutional endowment? By providing similarly traumatized infants with experimentally controlled environments, the third variable, constitution, could be isolated. Fajardo discovered that there are some infants for whom there are no good-enough, or empathic-enough mothers, that is, mothers who can effectively overcome their infants' developmental lags in self-organization. Infants who are deficient in self-regulating capacities and vulnerable to overstimulation need especially empathic mothers, and even then development is compromised. Her discussion provokes two questions for self-psychology: At what point in development does the selfobject concept pertain?; and, are selfobject phenomena relevant in normal development? Fajardo writes in relation to the more vulnerable premies' need for active soothing:

> Perhaps this more pronounced need for a particular environmental responsiveness in certain of our premies is germane to the concept of the selfobject: the vulnerable child, with the self in danger, is in need of a caretaker's selfobject function. The vulnerable infant is unable to maintain a phase appropriate cohesive self [p. 10].

One might infer, incorrectly I believe, that Fajardo is implying that the premie has a cohesive self and experiences selfobject functions. But Stern (1985) makes clear that such capacities are not phase appropriate in so young an infant, that during the first two months, the period of the emergent self, the infant is only beginning to form a sense of self; a core self is not yet achieved. Such a contention makes the selfobject concept in this early state equally questionable; the selfobject concept is closely linked to the development of the sense of self. If we stick to the idea that the selfobject function has meaning only as a subjective experience, it raises the question, Is so young an infant capable of anything approximating such an experience? Stern, who is most generous in ascribing a subjective world to the young infant, does not see the formulation of a sense of core self until at least two months. Thus, Stern provides us with a benchmark for postulating the capacity for appreciating the self-regulating other, which can be understood as one type of selfobject, a type that appears early in development and continues throughout the life cycle. Incidentally, Stern provides other benchmarks for selfobject function, such as a *self-attuning* other during *intersubjective* relatedness, which begins at seven months, and a *self-validating* other during *verbal* relatedness, beginning at 15 months. I think the answer to the first question posed, How soon is it valid to speak of selfobject function?, is that we must wait until a cohesive self is a possibility; that is, between two and six months of age. Moreover, for a fuller, richer selfobject experience, 15 to 18 months is a more reasonable time frame for its beginning.

But that leads us to the second, and much more far reaching, question, Does selfobject experience pertain to normal development? Fajardo appears to answer for herself, in the negative:

> . . . the experience of a selfobject is not essential to stimulate or propel the normal development of early infancy for the average or well-endowed child, in the average or better environment. But it is particularly relevant to the experience of infants who are either constitutionally vulnerable to disorganization or fragmentation, or are placed in danger of disorganization by an unempathic environment [p. 97–98].

This contention supports a definition of the selfobject as limited to subjectively perceived experiences with another utilized to shore up a *pathologically* faltering self, separating out the concept of the selfobject and selfobject experience for use only in explaining abnormality. Experiences in normal development with self-sustaining and self-augmenting others would be omitted from the selfobject definition. Two categories of experience with others required for self-augmentation would thus be delineated: the normal and the abnormal. I believe this position may be a response to Stern's persuasive argument that a normal phase of self-other undifferentiation, during the first six months of life, is not supported by observational data; therefore, he says, a selfobject concept that postulates fusion or lack of differentiation between self and object should not be conceptualized as an aspect of normal development, but, rather, as a pathological formation secondary to a faltering self. Stern argues:

Notions of a sense of a core self and the construction of normal self regulating others appears to be more in line with and useful to the general outlines of a theory of self psychology. This would replace the selfobject in normality with a self regulating other [p. 242].

Another way to remain consistent with Stern is to retain the concept of the selfobject in normal development as functioning to augment or shore up the self, and to see the differentiation or lack of differentiation between self and other as variable. This would make the self-regulating other of Stern's work a type of selfobject, along with the self-attuning other and the self-validating other.

Fajardo concludes that

constitutional factors may explain some limitations in what can be accomplished in a particular treatment situation, for instance, with chronically and pervasively anxious or overwhelmed patients, . . . [and may] lead to certain educative parameters in treatment [p. 99].

As she says, while an awareness of constitutional factors may seem academic owing to the focus in treatment on subjective experience, regardless of what etiological factors may be present, nevertheless such considerations are useful. I agree. I am convinced that the analyst's awareness of constitutional factors may help in formulating treatment strategies and in tempering analytic zeal. Above all, it facilitates empathic understanding of the patient's excruciating difficulties in mastering the anxiety producing situation.

Let me provide a brief illustration. This patient comes to mind because although not, strictly speaking, termed a premature infant at birth, she was born several weeks before term, had a low birthweight, and remained in the hospital for an extra week. I believe, however, that the more moderate trauma of her slight prematurity was overshadowed by the serious psychological pathology in her mother, which influenced her caretaking abilities. Moreover, and this is more to the point, there appeared to be a constitutional predisposition to poor self-regulation.

Patricia, now a 24-year-old law student, began treatment with me five years ago, following an unsuccessful attempt to attend college away from home, which experience led to intense depression, anxiety, and disorganization. She was hospitalized briefly, diagnosed as borderline, and was treated by a psychiatrist for about a year in intensive therapy, after which she decided that it was too difficult to be away from home and chose to attend college in Los Angeles.

She is the only child of divorced parents, the father powerful in his academic field, and the mother alcoholic, phobic, and considered a failure by her daughter. The early history of the patient includes a severe case of dysentery when she was two, and a traumatic episode of soiling at age three. Subsequently, she would have periodic bouts of anxiety related to a fear of becoming sick and being unable to find a bathroom, or experiencing endless and uncontrolled vomiting or diarrhea in a public restroom and being stuck forever, unable to leave. When she was in sixth grade, she suffered from school phobia for a year and remained at home. Patricia remembers her mother as always emotionally distant, depressed, and unavailable. For example, she remembers at age six having a tooth removed in a dentist's office and begging her mother to come in with her. Her mother refused, despite her pleas, saying she couldn't bear to see her in pain. Patricia's father, also distant, was openly demeaning of women. When he left Patricia's mother, Patricia felt deserted by him. Both parents became less valued in her eyes, and she felt less valued in theirs. In therapy with me, she found herself in the hands of someone whom she devalued and felt dismissive toward, consistent with her father's clear views of women. From the beginning, she was fearful of crying in front of me, terrified that I would be upset and unable to contain her, like her mother.

She soon developed a close friendship, and an almost nonexistent sexual relationship, with Robert, who functioned for her as a selfobject with both mirroring and idealizing features, and who served to displace the intensity of her transference need. Originally a friend and junior colleague of her father's and respected by him, Robert is highly gifted, but obsessive, passive, and somewhat effeminate. Patricia realized that Robert calmed, comforted, and reassured her with his unvarying availability and acceptance, but she was not aware of the extent that he served to allay her overwhelming anxiety, until, in an emotional confrontation, her father's true feelings of disparagement toward Robert emerged.

It was following this that an agoraphobia began in earnest. In addition, Patricia was forced to confront more directly her transference feelings toward me, much facilitating the therapeutic work. But, although during this productive period in therapy she was able to utilize repairative selfobject experiences, gain insight, and form a convincing life narrative, Patricia was still vulnerable to panic. Thus, while she came more fully to understand and master the trauma of being raised by her narcissistically damaged and damaging parents, the residual proneness to disorganizing affects required the use of psychopharmacological agents. The past history of self-regulatory difficulties in this patient, and her slow and difficult therapeutic course, can be most usefully conceptualized by invoking constitutional factors, in this case, a biochemical imbalance. Fajardo's data provide a scientific rationale for such therapeutic interventions, and I am indebted to her for her contribution.

Fajardo concludes by reminding us that some people, like my patient Patricia, do not easily, if ever, develop a robust self-regulatory ability; others also have dismal histories and unempathic environments throughout development and yet are highly responsive to treatment and can make surprising use of the therapeutic situation. I believe it is through the efforts of developmentalists such as Fajardo that we can gain an understanding of what creates the differences between these two categories of patients.

REFERENCES

Stern, D. N. (1985) *The Interpersonal World of the Infant.* New York: Basic Books.

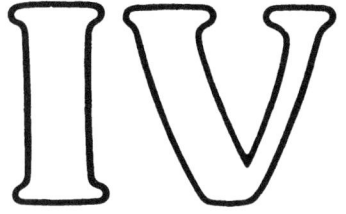

Clinical Papers

Chapter 8

Optimum Frustration: Structuralization and the Therapeutic Process

David M. Terman

This chapter reconsiders the psychoanalytic theory of structuralization—especially the centrality of frustration. I shall argue that the theoretical emphasis on frustration has neglected the importance and variety of pattern that is generated in transaction, in which a variety of responses and fulfillments play central roles in the construction of self experience, meaning and expectation.

In his last work, *How Does Analysis Cure?* (1984), Kohut again enshrined the concept of optimal frustration as central to the process of transmuting internalization. He asked the question, "Can abiding functions be acquired by the self without a preceding frustration, however tiny and/or fractionated from the side of the selfobject?" (p. 100). And he answered no. He detailed a three-step sequence: "1) need-activation and optimal frustration via 2) nonfulfillment of the need (abstinence) and 3) substitution of direct need fulfillment with the establishment of a bond of empathy between self and selfobject . . ." (p. 103). With the emphasis on frustration, Kohut put his concepts directly in line with classical theory and carefully divorced his theories and techniques from the onus of providing gratification.

I do not think I need to review the long and weighty reasons for the opprobrium in which the idea of gratification has been held. But since all impulses from which structure evolved were originally conceived by Freud to be sexual, gratification has meant something ranging from the regressive, antitherapeutic, or addictive to—in its most concrete and primitive form—the grossly unethical. So, the concept of frustration, in addition to its theoretical centrality, has acquired the quality of moral purity, if not righteousness.

Because of this, the exploration of those aspects of the therapeutic experience which are satisfying has been hampered. Further, our whole theory of structure formation—the acquisition of pattern and meaning—has been seriously skewed. (The clearest exception to this has been the excellent recent work of Bacal, whose contribution I discuss later.) In our exploration of the therapeutic process and structure formation, not only will we find other ways to conceptualize structure formation, but we shall also change or discard the concept of gratification insofar as it has connoted the satisfaction of erotic or erotically derived needs.

We are led to this reconsideration by two sources. The first, and more important, is that practice has not conformed well to theory. Reluctantly and increasingly, I have felt that changes in my patients occurred because of an understanding of the old and a creation of the new that arose from the experience in the analysis that had nothing to do with frustration. Often, but not always, interpretation or understandings or aspects of the analytic relationship itself answered—that is, satisfied—deeply held needs. It was the satisfaction of the needs that opened new paths and remade old ones. Some of the case reports in our literature have led me to the same conclusion.

The second source is the data from developmental studies. As investigators have become more sophisticated, their data appear more and more relevant to our own questions. Although we must always be careful about our use of their data—especially since some of the most systematic such studies concern the infant—we cannot help being struck by the complexity and variety of transactions they describe in which the child acquires its enduring regulatory, organizing, and affective patterns. It would indeed stretch our belief in the concept of frustrations-as-central-to-the acquisition of pattern, to see these structures arising and developing as the consequence of the absence or interruption of these transactions.

I consider both of these classes of data—the clinical and the developmental—in my discussion of structuralization, and I shall begin with the second, the developmental.

Lev Vygotsky, the Russian psychologist, was the first of the developmentalists to systematically explore the importance of environment in the creation of the child's conceptual world. His ideas about the acquisition of language stressed its interpersonal genesis. More generally, he saw all higher cognitive functions as originating in actual relations between people; for Vygotsky (1978), ''an interpersonal process is transformed into an intrapersonal one" (p. 57). For him, language and conceptual development grew out of the nature and process of communication. The structuralization of the mind grew out of human relationships and could not be understood apart from them.

Kenneth Kaye, a modern developmentalist, takes this position yet further. He (1982) discusses the difference between Vygotsky's understanding of development and Piaget's. Whereas Piaget's theories, like Freud's, stress development as "inside-out" (as the unfolding of innate, internally determined patterns), to use Kaye's distinction, Vygotsky's is "outside-in." Kaye, to his own surprise, finds that Vygotsky's ideas apply not only to childhood, during and after language acquisition, but to infancy as well. Kaye is even more emphatic about the importance of the parental role in creating and structuring the infant's mind. He sees the infant as an apprentice who is induced into a societal system by the goals and techniques of the parent. He finds "a great deal of asymmetry in the relations between parent and infant, so that the temporal structure that eventually becomes a true societal system will at first only have been created by the parent, making use of built-in regularities in infant behavior rather than actual cooperation or communication" (p. 53). Those structures which appeared to Piaget to evolve autonomously seem, for Kaye, to arise from the matrix *parental* goals and expectations. Speaking of the development of shared intentions, for example, a period beginning at two months, Kaye notes that the sharing begins as a "unilateral responsibility [of the parent]. . . . Adults guess at the intentions underlying infant's activity . . . parents have many ways of speaking for the child . . . what the parents are doing is integrating the new child into their already existing social system" (p. 66).

Kaye goes on: "By 8 months or so, the sharing of intentions has become a two-way process. The infant's schemes, differentiated *through experience in certain behavioral frames imposed by adult behavior,* allow him to anticipate the most likely direction of that behavior" (p. 67, italics added.) The infant goes on to a phase that Kaye calls shared memory and then to one of shared language. In all of these, Kaye notes, "the parents are constantly drawing the child forward into a more challenging apprenticeship, eventually a full partnership" (p. 68).

The parents "frame" the child's behavior; that is, they provide essential functions and regulations for the child. Kaye describes seven such frames: nurturant; protective; instrumental—the adult carries out what appears to be the child's intention, such as helping him get a toy beyond his reach; feedback, when the adult provides consequences of an action like prohibition or praise; modeling, in which the adult performs an action the child will imitate (often in the context of something the child is attempting himself); discourse, with the parent doing things to the child that have a predictable effect, for example, tickling, getting a response, and repeating, hence creating a kind of dialogue; and, finally, the memory frame, in which the parent remembers what the child likes and does not like and arranges important aspects of the child's world accordingly.

It is within these frames that the child begins to "take turns" and a dialogue evolves. Kaye's contention, again, is that this dialogue is virtually induced by the parent. The parent has the memory, expectations, and skills and by virtue of these moves the child into transactions that eventually create a shared symbolic system and a structure of goals and intentions. Kaye's analysis and description of a dialogue with a two year old illustrates the process. In a situation in which a mother and child are looking at a picture book, the "conversation" is recorded and analyzed. It goes like this (p. 100):

Mother	Child
1. (Points to picture)	
What is that one? (M)	2. Kitty cat. (R)
3. Well, what is it? (RM)	4. Kitty cat. (R)
5. Well, I know there's a	6. Huh? (RM)
kitty in it; what's he	
in? (RM)	
7. What's he riding in? (RM)	8. Airplane. (R)
9. Right. (R)	
10. (Turns page) (U)	

Most of the mother's participation involves what Kaye calls "mands" (M). A mand is an act that demands a response (R): a question or a request or pointing. It is by virtue of the mands that the child responds and a sequence develops. The existence and nature of the sequences depend on the mother's framing of the situation. She creates the structure of a dialogue. Kaye notes:

> So the child does not have the problem, as was once thought, of constructing a knowledge of his parents' language from a corpus of overheard speech. Instead he is plunged into ongoing discourse on topics very largely selected by his own interests. His meanings are interpreted, expressed and expiated upon almost before he really means anything at all. . . . the social structure, the discourse itself, is not mastered by children before they go on to the specifics of their parents' syntax and semantics. Adults will create and maintain the discourse structure for them, thus teaching them how to participate in that structure and *eventually take it over as their own* [p. 103].

The active creation of context results in the child's assimilating and then accommodating—taking in and, as a result, changing—the schemas, the patterns, with which he or she organizes the world. The changing and growth of patterns occur in the context of intense interaction. The *interaction*, not the spaces between the interactions, changes and structures. It is not the *loss* of the transaction, but rather its *presence* that structures.

The structure that emerges—the capacity to understand the labels attached to things and the capacity to take turns (among the many capacities generated in this dialogue)—would be inconceivable without the presence of these transactions. One could argue that it is only by giving the child space/time to absorb such experiences that permanent alteration in the child's mental organization is possible. But it stretches credulity to maintain that the *withholding*, or *delay*, of such transactions is *the* essential step in development of the structures that accrue from them. Further, to concentrate on a hypothetical delay to the neglect of the transaction misses the central areas of experience without which there can be nothing.

Daniel Stern, a psychoanalytic developmentalist, underlines the importance of the parent in helping to create what he calls self. Stern (1985) describes four phases of development of the self that take place during the first two years of life. These are the sense of emerging self, the sense of core self, the sense of subjective self, and the sense of a verbal self. Central to the construction of pattern is the concept of RIG—Representation of Interactions that have been Generalized. Stern finds evidence that self and other are distinguished very early (a finding that, I believe, will necessitate the revision of some of our notions of the nature of early self development) but that the "other" does, indeed, play a crucial role in the function of the self. Indeed, the essential regulatory role of the experience of the selfobject is confirmed and amplied by Stern's (1985) work.

For example, the parent plays a central part in the establishment and maintenance of the core self. This is defined as a sense of agency, coherence, affectivity, and history. It is an experiential, not a cognitive, construct. In that construction, the contouring of excitation is an important dimension, and the vignette of Eric is illustrative.

> Eric is a somewhat bland infant compared with his more affectively intense mother, but both are perfectly normal. His mother constantly likes to see him more excited, more expressive and demonstrative about feelings, and more avidly curious about the world. When Eric does show some excitement about something, his mother adroitly joins in and encourages, even intensifies, the experience a little—usually successfully—so that Eric experiences a higher level of excitement than he would alone. . . . Eric's self-experience or higher-than-usual excitement is, in fact, large-

ly achieved and regulated by his mother's behavior. His experience of his own higher levels of excitement occurs only in the lived episodes in which her augmentary antics are a crucial attribute. She thus becomes for him a self-excitement-regulating other. Eric's self-experience of high positive excitement never occurs unless mother is there participating in it. Specific episodes coalesce to form a RIG [p. 193].

This vignette is consistent with what we call a selfobject—probably a mirroring selfobject. The mother is an integral part of the psychological regulation of the child. How does the pattern become established here? By repetition. The participation of the mother in the child's excitement and her repeated augmentation of it eventually lead to the establishment of an inner state that can be reevoked and with which the world is experienced. Repetition and participation, *not absence*, lay down governing patterns.

The elements of repetition and participation are even more evident in the process Stern calls "attunement," which comes a little later, when the child is about nine months. The mother responds to the child by matching, cross-modally, the feeling state of the child. This is a crucial phenomenon in its own right, for, Stern holds, this kind of experience shifts attention away from simple external behavior to "what is behind the behavior, to the quality of feeling that is being shared" (p. 142). Hence attunement is a way of perceiving or sharing internal states.

The shaping, molding, and structuring of internal states may then occur by way of the vicissitudes of attunement. By selectively attuning, for example, the parent underlines and selects some experiences over others. As Stern notes:

> Parents have to make a choice, mostly out of awareness, about what to attune to, given that the infant provides almost every kind of feeling state. . . . This process of creating an intergenerational template is part of ordinary everyday transactions. . . . In being themselves, parents inevitably exert some degree of selective bias in their attunement behaviors and in doing so they create a template for the infant's sharable interpersonal world [p. 208].

II

Both the data and the thought of these developmentalists show us over and over and in many contexts that the creation of pattern occurs in significant transactions. And pattern is structure. Hence the focus of our inquiry shifts. We were interested in internalization as the sine qua non of structure formation; but as we examine the issue more close-ly, we see that the essential question is not so much internalization, but creation. What makes the pattern in the first place? The experience itself seems to make the pattern. The formation of structure seems not to be a two-step process. That is, it is not something that happens and then is separately transposed inside. Rather the participation itself changes the child's inner construction.

Freud's abandonment of the seduction hypothesis directed him to the vicissitudes of the *internal* construction of pattern and meaning—i.e. fantasy. With the emphasis on both internal generation of mean-ing and its accrual through frustration or loss, our attention has been drawn from the contextual *creation* of pattern in transaction. The con-cept of the selfobject has, of course, turned our attention back to these transactions. For self is maintained, generated, brought into existence, shaped in the experience of selfobject.

Let us turn now to some clinical data to examine these ideas fur-ther. If we look at the vicissitudes of the mirror transference, for ex-ample, we will see that we participate in the formation of important aspects of the patient's experience of self by our interpretations, by the framework of psychological values with which our interpretations are given, and by our therapeutic stance in general.

I have chosen to look at a fragment of one of the cases in the case-book (Goldberg, 1978) to illustrate these issues. It is the case of Mr. E. He was a 26-year-old married man who presented symptoms of anger with his wife, boredom, sensitivity to slights, and a work inhi-bition. His history included his having been born prematurely to a mother who was depressed and ill at his birth and experienced a progressive illness until her death when he was 15.

The analysis, begun after several months of psychotherapy, centered on a mirror transference in which exhibitionistic impulses and wishes for a variety of responses were expectably engaged and stimulated. Weekend separations and vacations also played an important role in his feelings of coherence and his level of energy. An important voyeuristic perversion emerged only after the analysis was underway, and the symptom became part of the process in response to the sepa-ration from the analyst. The patient revealed the symptom during the hour after he had given his analyst a Christmas card. The analyst had taken it and said thank you. The patient expressed gratitude that the analyst didn't interpret it. He said that he felt that it would have reduced the "genuineness of my behavior." In the next hour, he first told the analyst about his peeping at penises in men's bathrooms.

This sequence was paradigmatic for important aspects of the ana-lytic process. In this exchange, it was the patient's experience of the analyst as accepting that permitted a deepening of the process—the patient was first able to tell of an important symptom and begin engaging it and his underlying needs more deeply with the analyst. In this instance the participation—the analyst's act of acceptance—led not to a structural change, but to a deepening of the process rather than to a defensive repression of his underlying needs.

Exhibitionistic wishes became mobilized shortly thereafter in a dream in which the patient was in the analytic room, but elevated in the center of the couch. At the same time he began to feel depressed during the weekend separations, and his voyeuristic perversion was enacted. In one poignant Monday hour he reported frequenting men's rooms. The analyst (Goldberg, 1978) said, "He reported a sense of feeling bizarre." In a desolate voice, the patient reported having spent the time he was not in men's rooms painting empty chairs in his apartment. Suddenly he shouted, "I demand to know what you are thinking. You think I'm psychotic, don't you?" The analyst replied, "I think you must have been very lonely." The patient then burst out crying and said, when he recovered himself a bit, "That was the first time anyone ever realized that." He paused and added, "and I think that includes me" (p. 271).

Here was an interpretation that obviously had enormous immediate impact, and as one reads the case one sees repeated instances of this kind together with profound structural changes in the patient. What was the meaning of this kind of intervention? It certainly made the patient aware of a feeling that had been previously unavailable to him. Perhaps it made the experience into an affect and hence more symbolically transformable. But what seemed most important to the patient was the fact of being understood. His inner state was accurately perceived and accepted. He experienced himself as the center of the analyst's attention (as indeed he was). By implicitly understanding the patient's need for the analyst and explicitly noting the loneliness, the analyst helped create an experience in which the patient did not feel alone or unattended. This occurred in the context of the revival of the experience of aloneness and lack of investment (weekend separation). I contend that the building of structure, the acquisition of pattern, occurred by virtue of the analyst's response, understanding; and the creation of that new pattern followed from the experience of the understanding and was not created by the absence of understanding. The internalization was implicit in, dependent on the construction—the presence of the understanding.

But one can raise an immediate objection. Was it not, after all, the *frustration*, the weekend separation, that was integral to the experience? Does this not follow Kohut's formulation, as we stated it in the beginning, that is, need activation and optimal frustration via nonfulfillment of the need and substitution of direct need fulfillment with the bond of empathy. . . ? The separation functioned as the frustration of the need, and the interpretation of loneliness constituted the empathic bond. If one looks at it that way, what was the nature of the archaic need consistent with this explanation? Was it the need to be with the parent physically all the time? If it were that, the formulation would fit, at least in the sense that something else was offered for it. But that is a rather concrete understanding of the nature of the need. Rather the patient needed the analyst's interest and investment and acceptance. These were certainly absent as far as the patient was concerned, at least over the weekend. But the interpretation did not then *substitute* for the fulfillment of the need; the interpretation satisfied the need. If the requirement was interest and investment, being the center of the analyst's attention, the need has been met. Hence one could say that frustration was, indeed, the stimulus for the subsequent satisfaction, but the satisfaction was not a substitute.

The central question still remains: What is responsible for the creation of pattern? Could the experience of analyst-as-understanding-paying-attention and patient-feeling-valued (or cohesive) exist without the analyst's interpretation? No. Could it have occurred without the antecedent frustration? It seems not. Is the enduring quality of that experience dependent on the antecedent or subsequent-absence of the experience? No. I submit that such absences or interruptions provide the occasion for the experience of the analyst-as-understanding. It is the *repetition* of the *presence* that builds new structure. (The repetition of the *absence* reevokes the old patterns.) And this is much of the reason for and substance of the working through.

In many subsequent transactions, one sees more clearly the importance of the experience of the analyst as understanding and sustaining as *longings* for consistent responsiveness were mobilized without antecedent frustration. The patient had two homosexual dreams with overt and disguised transference manifestations after several frustrations and rejections from women. The patient became both aware of, and embarrassed by, the homosexual wishes for the analyst. The analyst interpreted them in a genetic context—a turning to the father after a disappointment with the mother.

The patient then had a dream that he reported the next day. His chairman had looked at several reports he had done and said, "I'll take it down to the bindery." The analyst reported the following:

> He associated to psychoanalysis and how it had helped him—that he now understood the "authority" of his experiences. He was not sure

what he meant by that, but thought of a leader holding the diverse elements of a country together. "Here [referring to the analysis] both fact and fantasy are treated with respect. That is a comfort to me—you accept what I said about my sexual behavior." He felt that this made him less of a stranger to himself and that he felt less lonely as he saw that "there is understanding to be had. You are helpful because you are not threatened by my needs" [p. 276].

In this instance, it is more clear that the analyst's understanding, and, if anything, facilitation, of the patient's yearnings are the heart of the patient's experience. The stimulus for the yearnings is not a frustration by the analyst. Neither the interpretation nor its effect are frustrating. The patient felt bound together—more cohesive—as the result of both. He felt the analyst was not threatened by his needs for him. He could experience, express, and find satisfaction of many levels of need. Surely the need for understanding his feelings and the awareness of, and interest in, his inner state was amply fulfilled. And this was at the same level as the childhood experience. The inner experience and the transactions establishing them are not so different from what the child most centrally needs.

The feeling that the analyst was not threatened, that he accepted the patient's needs, may also serve a regulatory, integrative function that had been warded off or not yet given coherent form. This analytic act changes existing structure or creates structure anew—that is, it helps form a pattern of experience of self-acceptance, or self-existence. And it is the presence of the act that creates pattern. Will it then be internalized? I think it is being internalized in the making.

The patient's experience of acceptance, and the analyst's communicating acceptance through his interpretations, seem to be an essential part of the patient's construction and reconstruction of himself.

The vacation at some point after this episode produced a sense of impending fragmentation. The analyst reports: "He reported feeling decrepit, complained he was lacking compared to others. He thought of lizards, rats and a guillotine. He could actually see heads rolling and hear the squish of dead bugs on the pavement" (p. 276). The analyst called attention to his upcoming vacation, to which the patient responded with embarrassment over his wishing for the presence of the analyst. His awareness of the feeling, and, again, of the analyst's understanding of it, seemed to lead to a reintegration and further recall of, and connection with, his mother's deterioration and death.

Here the impending absence—the prospective vacation—restimulated the experience of loss of attention and loss of self; but after the interpretation of his feeling and the reintegration of the interpretation, the patient had further access to the memory and affect around his mother's deterioration. Something had changed in the patient—both the control of the regression and the useful reexperience of the past—that permitted a reproduction of the old experience in a new framework. (This is nothing new, of course. We all see this every day in every functioning analysis. Indeed, the whole analytic process is viewed this way.) I contend that the interpretation here supplied exactly what the patient was missing in reliving the past: the alive, understanding presence. It did so also by virtue of the structure that had already begun to grow and consolidate—a self, if you will, that was vital, continuous, even lovable—and acquired in the experience of the analyst's interpretations, presence, and acceptance.

Certainly vacations and weekends, in this case, provided the opportunity to reexperience aspects of the past, but I am maintaining that the reintegration and new integration around those periods depended on understanding and responses that were not substantially different from what was required in the past, and that the reformation of the old and formation of the new patterns grew out of the fulfillment of the requirements, not their frustrations.

III

There are obvious and enormous differences between development and the therapeutic situation. First, as I noted, the developmental data to which I have referred are from infants under two. Stern (1985) makes the interesting assumption that such infants mainly experience reality. He writes, "Their subjective experiences suffer no distortion by virtue of wishes or defenses, but only those made inevitable by perceptual or cognitive immaturity or overgeneralization (p. 255). Hence, the complexity of acquired inner structure and the processing of experience by such a more complex structure are missing. Second, the situation of newly developing structure—of laying down for the first time—is, of course, quite different from the therapeutic encounter with, and mobilization of, preexisting structure. The raison d'etre of the transference is the reevolution of such preexisting and otherwise inaccessible structure. Indeed, the way the patient experiences us as participating is already determined by such preexisting structure.

Yet the core of *change* of that structure—or the creation of a new structure, the resolution of the transference—always entails an experience of the analyst that is different from the past. Classically, this has meant only a change in the perception of the analyst because of the change in inner organization effected by the altered defensive structure—that is, it has been viewed as an internal change from purely internal factors. The concept of the selfobject, however, has permitted us to examine the therapeutic process and systematically explore the role and meaning of our responses in the genesis and change of those inner structures. And when we turn to these phenomena and examine them, the parallels are suggestive, even striking.

We do not "frame" precisely the way Kaye (1982) observes in the parent-child relationship. We do not, for example, supply memory or effect the various cognitive functions; we do not create a cognitive dialogue. However, we do participate in an *affective dialogue* in which the inner structure that we call self changes or emerges. In the case described, the analyst's interest, investment, understanding and acceptance—especially of the patient's longings for precisely those qualities from the analyst—constituted the responses in a dialogue in which the analyst was an essential member and in which the experience of a whole, alive, and lovable self emerged. i suspect the process is not unlike Stern's RIG—representation of interactions that have been generalized. Often in relation to the old RIG—the experience of the depleted mother and the dying weak self—the new or changed self is created. But it is also created anew as in the episode in which the longings for the analyst were by implication validated and accepted. That was a new opportunity in which a new experience of self was generated. The analogy, if not homology, between this process and Stern's (1985) description of the development of a state of self-excitement in Eric, is highly suggestive.

A theory of structure formation that emphasizes our participation is indicated. Socarides and Stolorow (1984/85) have pointed to the same issue. Confining their concerns to cases of early selfobject failure, they postulate that "the central curative element may be formed in the selfobject transference bond itself" (p. 112). It is the intactness of the selfobject tie that permits the resumption of growth on these cases. Similarly, in discussing the metabolism of depressive affect, they shift the emphasis of the mechanism of change from optimum frustration to the centrality of affect attunement.

Bacal (1985) has offered the term "optimal responsiveness" to emphasize the appropriate ways the analyst can respond in accordance with the patient's phase-appropriate and individually specific requirements for growth or repair. This felicitous term emphasizes the necessity for participation and response in the formation of pattern, and helps us look beyond the narrow confines of the concept of frustration to consider a much richer and broader spectrum of experience—both in development and the therapeutic process.

The emphasis on participation in the formation of pattern is not to deny that frustration also creates pattern. It does. Further, not all participation leads to adaptive, harmonious pattern; some leads to distorted, maladaptive structure. And, in fact, more of the distortions of structure are due to mismatches of responses of many sorts than are due to nonresponse. But to make frustration the central mechanism of pattern creation distracts our attention from the variety and significance of an enormous spectrum of transaction that is so far suggested in both developmental and therapeutic fields.

Bacal (1985) states, "We cannot assume that all internalizing processes occur through frustration. In a good enough situation, for example, identification and assimilation occur" (p. 22). I would be more emphatic. I suspect that internalization and structure formation have little to do with frustration, and I do not think identification and assimilation quite account for the power and pervasiveness of a system of communication, affective dialogue, in which pattern is generated.

I suggest the phrase "dialogue of construction" to characterize this process of structure. The doing is the making. The dialogue is the structure. The repetition—not the absence or interruption—creates the enduring pattern.

This is the essential stuff of which we are made—and remade. And this is what we must continue to study.

REFERENCES

Bacal, H. (1985), Optimal responsiveness and the therapeutic process. In: *Progress in Self Psychology*, Vol. 1, ed. A. Goldberg. New York: Guilford Press.

Goldberg, A., ed. (1978), *The Psychology of the Self: A Casebook*. New York: International Universities Press.

Kaye, K. (1982), *The Mental and Social Life of Babies*. Chicago, IL: University of Chicago Press.

Kohut, H. (1984/5), *How Does Analysis Cure?* Chicago, IL: University of Chicago Press.

Socarides, D. & Stolorow, R. (1987), affect and selfobjects. *Annual of Psychoanalysis*, Vol. 12-13. New York: International Universities Press.

Stern, D. (1985), *The Interpersonal World of the Infant*. New York: Basic Books.

Vygotsky, L. S. (1978), *Mind in Society*. Cambridge, MA: Harvard University Press.

Chapter 9

Reflections on "Optimum Frustration"

Howard A. Bacal

My discussion of Terman's chapter can be brief, since he has amply affirmed my view that the concept of optimal frustration is not relevant to a self-psychological perspective on theory or practice in psychoanalysis (Bacal, 1985). My conceptualization of what is therapeutic, or curative, includes elements similar to his, and I will review this shortly.

Terman has in particular drawn attention to developmental studies by Vygotsky, Kaye, and Stern, which lend weight to the view that it is repeated participation by significant adult figures in constructive cognitive activity and affective attunement with the child that shapes, molds, and structures his internal states. These studies, in effect, call into question the notion of optimal frustration as a positive factor in psychological growth. I shall not comment further on them except to recognize that they support my contention that it is the *optimal responsiveness* to the needs and unique characteristics of the child by his caretakers that will determine healthy self-development.

Terman offers an interesting hypothesis about the creation of structure, which he bases on the repeated demonstration by these developmentalists that "the creation of pattern occurs in significant transactions" (this volume, p. 118). He suggests that, insofar as pattern can be regarded as structure, the notion of internalization may be irrelevant to the formation of structure, since it is the experience of the significant transaction itself that makes the pattern that is sufficient for the creation of structure. As Terman puts it, ''It is not something that happens and then is separately transposed inside. Rather the participation itself changes the child's inner construction'' (this volume, p. 119). This, of course, calls into question the relevance of the theory of *transmuting internalization via optimal frustration* for the laying down of structure, for personal growth, and for analytic cure. In short, the experience of optimal responsiveness (Bacal, 1985) may be sufficient. Terman suggests we use the phrase *dialogue of construction* for the process by which structure is formed. I welcome this term, as it underscores the object-relational, or interactional aspect of the process of personal development. Perhaps we could regard the two terms as complementary: The patient's experience of the analyst's optimal responsiveness is an indication that a dialogue of construction is taking place.

A person becomes a patient if, as a child, he did not have this experience with significant figures. Carrying his unhappiness in one hand and his hopes in another, he will seek responses from his therapist that will be optimal for the treatment of his illness and for a resumption of his emotional growth. I will summarize here my view of the therapeutic process in psychoanalysis.

The patient's expectations from and reactions to his therapist are determined both by previously negatively charged experience and by hopeful anticipation that the therapist will treat him differently. As therapy proceeds, the validity of both these attitudes will, to varying degrees, be confirmed. While they are often present as a complex mix, for purposes of study they can usefully be considered separately.

The recurring experience of the patient's early, negatively tinged relationships by either patient or analyst in relation to each other is not only inevitable, but is diagnostically and often therapeutically useful. The experience by the patient that the analyst is acting like the offending or frustrating nuclear figure, or even harboring attitudes toward him that are similar to theirs, or the realization by the analyst that he is doing so, offers valuable opportunities for both participants to understand and work through privations or disruptions of selfobject functioning, to the therapeutic benefit of the patient (and, incidentally, sometimes to some extent, of the analyst as well). However, none of these transference and countertransference experiences should be termed an optimal frustration, since there is nothing inherent in them that leads to psychological growth. Rather, it is a case of the analyst or the patient experiencing the other, for a time, as not optimally responsive. The same tasks—understanding and working through the patient's sense of chronic or recurring disruption of selfobject functioning in relation to significant nuclear figures as well as to figures in the patient's current life—are engaged in virtually every session when, for the most part, these tensions are not experienced between patient and analyst. In other words, in an ordinary, good-enough analysis, the experience of optimal responsiveness is the prevalent one. And, once again, it should be recognized that this is the case for both analyst and analysand; that is, optimal responsiveness will be a mutual experience, its antithesis being, in effect, "transference" and "countertransference," as we generally use these terms clinically.

While transference is usually defined as the patient's experience of his relationship with the analyst as determined by infantile experience, and countertransference as the totality of the analyst's reactions to them, in practice these terms designate not the total spectrum of experience, but those of the patient's and analyst's reactions to each other that are problematic. The patient's repetitive transferences and the analyst's repetitive countertransferences (repetitive in the sense that they repeat early problematic experiences) must be contrasted with what I have called the creative aspects of transference—the patient's experience of the analyst as a figure with whom a different or even new scenario might unfold or is already unfolding, and the analyst's constructive responses to them. This "positive" transference, as I have now described it is, I submit, what self psychology regards as selfobject transference, and the counterpart in the analyst is what I have earlier described as optimal responsiveness.[1] Thus, while the emergence of an archaic selfobject transference in analysis is symptomatic of a failure in early self-selfobject relationships, it is not only an expression of that failure. It is also an expression of the experience of that failure being redressed. Put in another way, the experience by the patient of the analyst's optimal responsiveness is the enabling factor for the experience and establishment of the selfobject transference. To what extent antecedent childhood selfobject experience is a precondition for the evolution and establishment of the selfobject transference in analysis is another important issue, but I shall not address this now.

I also agree with Terman that the interpretation that makes the patient feel understood is tantamount to the provision of what was missing in the past that contributed to the negative self-state, namely, "the alive, understanding presence"—in my language, the experience of optimal responsiveness. It is instructive to study analytic situations when this does not happen. In my initial communication (Bacal, 1985), I did not provide examples of interpretations that constitute optimal

---

[1]This could be termed, in parallel, selfobject countertransference, but it might lead to some confusion with so-called narcissistic countertransference, a problematic reaction in the analyst to the patient's selfobject needs toward him.

responsiveness simply because interpretations that appear effective are part and parcel of an analysis that is moving along satisfactorily and therefore would not serve as a demonstration of my proposition that a good interpretation is only one component of the analyst's optimal responsiveness (and, I suggest, possibly not even the most therapeutic one). I chose, rather, to illustrate my view with a clinical example that seemed to require a different order of optimal responsiveness. When interpretations persistently fail to provide this experience for the patient (as they did in that case), then apart from the possibility that the interpretations may be wrong, the likelihood of traumatic frustration in the patient's early childhood must be considered (p. 208). In these instances, the patient will require something out of the ordinary from the analyst in order to feel understood by him, something that the analyst may regard as out of order; a change of demeanor or attitude, perhaps some action, such as the acceptance of a gift, an alteration of fees or appointment time. The analyst may or may not be willing and/or able to provide them. It is as if the patient is now saying to the analyst, "Show me. *Be* who I need you to be, don't just interpret it." If the analyst cannot find a way to respond optimally to this appeal, the patient may continue and even intensify "acting-in" or may surface from the regression and accept the limitations of analysis for himself, at least with that analyst.

In effect, I am suggesting that the limitations of optimal responsiveness are determined by the effect on the analyst of the interacting self-object needs of both participants in the analytic process—that is, between that particular patient and that particular analyst—especially when the patient is in a deeply regressed state in the transference. It is at these times more than any other that the vulnerabilities of the patient may resonate with comparable ones in the analyst and strain his capacity to continue to respond optimally to his patient. To put this in another way, I believe that a closer study of this perspective on the therapeutic process may help us to understand better why "benign" regressions sometimes become "malignant."

Moreover, apart from the beneficial effect of the analyst's noninterpretive, optimal responsiveness that he provides his patient in regressive states, there is considerable noninterpretive, optimal responsiveness in the course of everyday analytic work—sometimes transitory but sometimes quite prevalent—that is of significant therapeutic benefit. Most analysts know in their heart that this is a crucially therapeutic aspect of all analyses much of the time. But they seldom talk about it, and it is almost never written about, unless its absence produces significant dissonance between patient and analyst, in which case providing it is regarded as a "parameter" and thus not properly psychoanalytic. Is this because of a tacit belief that this properly belongs to the "art" of psychoanalytic therapy and any attempt at a scientific consideration of it is not only fruitless but would undermine its effectiveness? Or is it mainly because we are uneasy about looking too closely at what we are doing for fear of being unable to justify it in the light of existing theory or according to how we have been trained? I submit that this area constitutes another frontier for psychoanalytic study. While this may stir anxieties to which few wish to expose themselves, I believe that the therapeutic rewards would justify the difficulties of the investigation.

REFERENCES

Bacal, H. (1985), Optimal responsiveness and the therapeutic process. In: *Progress in Self Psychology*, Vol. 1, ed. A. Goldberg. New York: Guilford Press, pp. 202–226.

Chapter 10

A Case of Intractable Depression

Bernard Brandchaft

Heinz Kohut's last paper (1982), written shortly before his death, summarized some of his most important differences with classical psychoanalysis and constituted his own legacy to succeeding generations of psychoanalysts. He had arrived at this point, painfully but inexorably, by his persistent dissatisfaction with the clinical results of the application of classical theories of development and pathogenesis and by his return, 25 years earlier, to the "field-defining observational stance of introspection and empathy " (p. 402).

In particular, Kohut took passionate issue with the concepts of intrapsychic conflict that have continued to provide the foundations for traditional psychoanalytic theories and practice. It was a tragic mistake, he insisted, to continue to treat people as if their essence were defined by a lifelong struggle between drives and the civilizing influences of their social environment as embodied in the superego. Error was compounded by the tendency of psychoanalysts to view their patients who fail to respond or who respond negatively to psychoanalytic attempts to understand and treat them from this perspective as "resisting therapeutic analysis because of unwillingness or inability to tame their aggressive/destructive wishes" that characteristically led them to become engaged in wars and self-destruction (p. 402).

To the classical view Kohut counterposed his own. The essence of man, he wrote, resided in his resourceful striving to preserve and unfold "his innermost self, *battling against external and internal obstacles to its unfolding*" (italics added) and his developmental course was shaped by his lifelong attempt, never quite successful, "to realize the program laid down in his depth during the span of his life" (p. 403). These contrasting views Kohut encapsulated, as he had done in earlier works, as "Guilty Man" or "Tragic Man."

Kohut went on in this paper to argue specifically that the intergenerational conflict of the Oedipus triangle and its resolution by renunciation of (presumably) pathogenic impulses or childhood claims was not central to normal development, as generations of analysts had come to accept. Instead, Kohut insisted as his own life was drawing to a close, "It is support for the succeeding generation...that is normal and human, [rather than] intergenerational strife and mutual wishes to kill and to destroy" (p. 404), however frequently the latter are to be found. It is only when the parent whose self is not normal, healthy, cohesive, vigorous and harmonious reacts with "seductiveness and competitiveness, rather than pride and affection...to the child's exhiliarated move toward a greater degree of assertiveness, generosity and affection" that the conflictful situation develops. This conflictful situation Kohut described as one of hostility and lust, and he referred to these as "break-up products" of the disintegration of the "newly constituted assertive affectionate self of the child" (p. 404).

In an earlier work (1977), Kohut spoke of a "pivotal point...(in) late middle age when nearing the ultimate decline, we ask ourselves whether we have been true to our innermost design" (p. 241). This was a

> time of utmost hopelessness for some, of utter lethargy...which overtakes those who feel that they have failed and cannot remedy the failure in the time and with the energies still at their disposal. The suicides of this period are not the expression of a punitive superego, but a remedial act—the wish to wipe out the unbearable...mortification...imposed by the ultimate recognition of a failure of all-encompassing magnitude. [p. 241]

Although in these passages Kohut established the observational basis for a developmental psychology of the self that encompasses both deficit and conflict, he stopped short of delineating the "internal and external obstacles" to the unfolding of the intrinsic program of the child's self, and that underlay the depression of all-encompassing failure to which he referred. The psychic conflicts that arise as sequellae of parental opposition to the child's attempt to crystallize a design true to his "innermost self" and in consequence of the parents' need for the child's repudiation of such singularity in his developmental

processes extend importantly beyond the conflicts of lust and hostility. They are contained within the panoply of pathological structural
distortions and misalignments that arise in derailments and miscarri-
ages of the developmental processes of self differentiation and self
articulation.

In recent papers, attempts have been made to focus on the genesis
and fate of intrapsychic conflict arising in the development of the self
(Brandchaft, 1986; Stolorow, Brandchaft, and Atwood, 1988; Atwood
and Stolorow, 1984).

> Every phase in a child's development is best conceptualized in terms
> of the unique psychological field constituted by the intersection of the
> child's evolving subjective universe with that of its caretakers . . . . Patho-
> genesis, from this intersubjective perspective, is understood in terms of
> severe disjunctions or asynchronies that occur between structures of sub-
> jectivity of parents and child, whereby the child's primary developmental
> needs do not meet with the requisite responsiveness from (self) objects.
> When the psychological organization of the parent cannot accomodate
> to the changing phase specific needs of the developing child, then the
> more malleable and vulnerable psychological structure of the child will
> accomodate to what is available. [Atwood and Stolorow, 1984, p. 69]

One of the possible outcomes, we suggested, was that the child may
develop symptoms in which sequestered nuclei of an archaic self are
preserved in conflict with, or in isolation from, the unresponsive selfobjects.

In the passages quoted earlier, Kohut drew attention to the fact that
the specific interplay between the child and his environment fur-
thers or hinders the cohesion of the self, as he also did in his final
book (1984, p. 562). There he also called for the detailed examination
of varieties of transferences in order to map out this interplay. Here
I wish to emphasize the importance of the varieties of specific parental responses that support or interfere with the second major developmental task—successful negotiation of the crucial sense of
individualized selfhood, its consolidation and elaboration in designs
of increasingly complex particularity, and the implications for anala-
gous selfobject transferences.

This, I believe, is the area of development in which environmental
failure most frequently results in inner conflict becoming structuralized. Such mishap occurs in the presence of an intersubjective context
in which central affect states associated with emerging and crystalliz-
ing individualized selfhood remain massively unresponded to or actively repudiated. The resultant psychic conflict involves not clashing
instincts or internalized objects but rather the frequently irreconcila-

ble motivations that the developmental course massively fit in with the needs of caretakers, on one hand, and, on the other, that developmental evolution remain firmly rooted in the vitalizing affective, generative, core of a self of one's own.

Attempts at resolution of this pervasive conflict can proceed in either of two directions. The child may attempt to preserve and protect this core of individualized vitality at the expense of object ties by determined nonconformism or rebellion. That is the path of isolation and ultimate estrangement. Alternatively, the child may abandon or fatally compromise his central strivings in order to maintain indispensable ties. That is the path of submission. Or the child may oscillate between these two.

Depression becomes the dominant affect in a person in whom such a conflict has become chronic and internalized. It signals the loss of hope when no synthesis can be found between intimate connectedness with important others and the pursuit of a program of individualized selfhood. When such despair occurs in middle age, as it did with the patient, Mr. N, who will presently be described, the conditions are set for the type of depression Kohut described so movingly in the passage quoted earlier.

The analytic setting, however, provides a context for the revival of an archaic tie in which development in this essential area can be resumed, even after a lifetime of conflict has resulted in utter hopelessness and lethargy. Such an attempt is always accompanied by an intense fear or conviction that the price for the analyst's help will once more involve a submissive distortion of self development.

Mr. N's treatment for severe and sometimes disabling depression has extended almost 15 years, interrupted and resumed three times during that period. He is a 50+ year old man of prodigious and diverse musical talents. Despite his undoubted gifts, success in the endeavor most precious to him, musical composition, has eluded him. His total repertory consists of seven works. Each composition was preceded and followed by an agonizing episode of depression, in which for long periods of time his creativity was paralyzed.

I noted over many years that severe depression invariably recurred following any success. This, together with Mr. N's pattern of relentless self-reproaches, led me for some time to conclude that his depression was rooted in a pathological superego and an unconscious sense of guilt. Although Mr. N seemed to concur in such explanations and provided an abundance of corroborative material, his hopelessness seemed to increase. Closer attention to the impact of these interpretations over a long period of time enabled me to recognize that my understanding had been faulty. These interpretations had conveyed to Mr. N. that I believed that there was some essential condition existing solely within him that was defeating him at every turn. They thus tended repetitively to reinforce his worst fears about himself. They failed to take into account how urgently he needed a tie with someone whom he could experience as willing to believe in his capabilities, in the purity of his purpose, and in his ultimate success, whatever the obstacles. The interpretations failed to recognize sufficiently how alone and disapproved of he had come to feel as a result of the interpretive stance which I had taken.

Mr. N's depression cleared sufficiently following the analysis of this situation for him to engage once more in creative endeavor, and he was able to complete an important work. He hoped that his being able to write signalled a complete disappearance of his depression. When the depression soon returned, it became a source of profound disappointment. No matter what the initial trigger might be in this period of time, the moment Mr. N began to feel depressed, a spiralling effect took place. For example, he might read in the newspaper of a fellow composer whose work was being played, and this was enough once more to remind him forcefully that his work was not being played and to start him on the road to despair. Once he began to feel dejected, Mr. N was confirmed in his belief that he was incurably flawed and forever doomed to depression, and he sank more deeply into this state. For hour after hour he would insist that it would never be different, that he could not be helped. This seemed absolutely logical and factual to him. He would cite repetitively that he had been depressed for as long as he could remember and, although he had tried many times, had found no help that lasted any substantial period of time. Perhaps, he would say, he could remember a few days of relief, but then the curtain had always descended once again. He had so grown to experience himself in this way that now when he felt momentarily relieved he would scrutinize his feelings expectantly, and once he could detect any letdown, the slide would get underway. This process was automatic, invariant, and not open to reflection—indications, I had come to recognize, of an unconscious organizing principle (Atwood and Stolorow, 1984, p. 36).

In this circumstance the analysis of the content of whatever had precipitated the depressive mood proved irrelevant, and it became clear that only the *context* into which it was being assimilated was relevant. I found myself then explaining how Mr. N experienced his depression. I stressed over and over again that the whole pattern and Mr. N's ultimate despair rested on his unquestioning acceptance that his fate had already been determined and his future foretold. For him there was to be no hope, no pleasure, and no career of his choosing, since what was most depressing for Mr. N was that his depression kept him absolutely from his life's work. I tried to introduce an alternative way of looking at his experience, namely that it was that conviction itself around which his experience repetitively became elaborated, not any inexorable fate. It was that which interfered with the recovery of his resilience whenever any setback might temporarily cast a pall on his sense of self and thus his mood and his outlook. He could not do anything to help himself when vagaries of his experience made him automatically feel that he was the victim of an incurable and global defect or were proof of an inexorable fate.

In his posture of seemingly complete hopelessness, Mr. N would also maintain over and over that the analysis was a failure and that it was an illusion to believe that anything could change. Frequently he would return to the assertion that I also felt, or would surely come to feel, hopeless about him and burdened by his hopelessness and inability to change. These feelings became even more unremitting when Mr. N was out of work for a prolonged period and was unable to pay anything toward his bill for treatment. Then he felt that everything I said was critical of him for continuing to feel depressed and an expression of how burdened I felt by him. In this connection, I came to appreciate that the function of holding of Mr. N's despair was crucial and that no arbitrary time period could be allotted for such experience, but that each depressive episode has its own internal and intersubjective dynamics. I realized that it was essential that my own hopeful attitude be sustained only by my absolute determination to do anything I could to understand his experience and my own and by Mr. N's showing up each day, no matter how hopeless or automatonlike, rather than by any attempt actively to alter his mood. I had to learn to monitor myself rigorously about this and to try to resist such urges when I could. Attempts to explain before Mr. N's subjective experience had been sufficiently elaborated were premature. They had the effect on him of being left alone in a short-circuited state. On the other hand, repeated experiences of shared affect, though without confirmation of his perspective, had the ultimate effect of establishing for Mr. N the necessary conditions for a feeling of safety and harmony that subsequently carried over into other affect states and made the understandings I could convey assimilable.

Mr. N proved extremely helpful to me in enabling me to sustain my attunement to his mood as it found its own baseline. Soon, after leaving particular sessions in which I had had little to say, he began to tell me the next day and sometimes as he got up to leave that he had felt better.

Thus, over a prolonged period, a milieu came to be established in which Mr. N could experience his depressive affects in all their intensity. His tendency to stifle those which had led previously to "dead" feelings was somewhat counteracted. The gradual assimilation of these feelings into a new relationship experience actually came to mark the beginning reinstatement of a traumatically compromised developmental process.

As Mr. N's conviction about his depressive experience subsided, he began to think more and more about his music. For a long time he would return obsessively to the fact that he had written so sparsely for all these years. "Now, when I'm my age, I'm going to start a career" he would say in a self-deprecatory way, "It's an illusion." And again sink into depression. "I can't be a composer, because a composer is somebody whose life is centered around music! I've been on vacation all my life. Nobody's ever heard of me. I'm a dilletante." And he would repeat this in endless variation for session after session. He would tell me that he had not listened to music for years and that he avoided going to concerts. Earlier, when Mr. N had been absolutely paralyzed creatively by his depression, he would return frequently to the statement that if he could only give up his delusion that he was a composer, he could escape from the agony that was his everyday lot. Then he would go on to make a convincing case that his illness consisted of his stubbornness in holding on to his desire to do something for which he was clearly unsuited. At the time, I did not recognize the conflictful and reactive nature of these protestations. I had emphasized his inability to move in *any* direction that would offer him relief from suffering, pointing to what appeared to be the deepest element of his character, a pathological need to suffer. Only gradually did I come to understand that Mr. N experienced my presumably neutral stance as a vote of no confidence in him. This became clearer as he began more openly to tell me that nobody had ever expected anything of him. When he was a child, and his mother would complain about him failing in school or giving her a hard time, his father would say "That's him— Ach, what do you expect?" He had always disappointed everyone in everything, he felt, so they learned not to expect anything. Since nobody really expected him to amount to anything, he could never sustain any incongruent expectation of himself.

Actually, seen from a different vantage point, Mr. N's gifts and achievements were prodigious in the face of the overwhelming obstacles that had been placed in his path. To appreciate more fully the creative talent Mr. N kept hidden, it was necessary to recognize and overcome my own fear of being disappointed in him if he persisted in his creative endeavor and of being responsible for having encouraged him. I was able to alter my stance so as to stress more consistently my understanding of the intensity of his anxieties that led him to wish that he could abandon his course. The psychological impediments in his path then became the focus of our investigation, and this strengthened his determination to compose. Subsequently it emerged that giving up his lifelong pursuit, whatever his age, would mean psychological death to him and that only if he felt supported in the attempt to understand and surmount the obstacles could he persist in his own struggle to crystallize a design of his own.

Two severe setbacks due to physical ailments occurred subsequently. The first happened about two and a half years before the sessions I will describe. It took several months for him to recover from its physical effects. The serious psychological complications took longer to resolve because he regarded the illness also as an act of fate, yet another, final, irrefutable proof that success, happiness, and the possibility of a unique life form were not for him. In the sessions that followed this first illness, Mr. N would sink relentlessly into a state of complete absorption with his victimhood. It took some time before he gradually recognized that there was something extremely appealing and comforting to him about this pull. Although his mother had been extremely intolerant of his feelings and reacted to his depressions generally as burdensome and damaging, it was different with sickness or physical injury. These states could consistently evoke her compassion. "Poor Tommy" she would intone characteristically, "He never gets a break!" Sometimes, when he would have a nosebleed or a severe stomach ache, she would minister to him in perfect attunement with a state she knew so well. "Well what do you expect?" she would say consolingly, as if the expectation of anything good was a symptom of an idiotic or disordered mind, "It's just the luck of the N's!"

Mr. N could not remember being able to elicit any similarly reliable interest or enthusiasm from her for any achievement of his own. And so it came to be that whenever he resurrected any enthusiasm in his life's work, it was invariably accompanied by an increasing sense of isolation and estrangement. He could only escape from this by reestablishing the more familiar sense of himself as victim. The role of his father was consistently to disparage as pretentious illusions the boy's dreams for himself, and so to increase N's sense of isolation when he embarked on a goal of his own.

As he recovered from this illness, Mr. N came to realize how his underlying conviction that he had been born to lose itself had contributed to the course his life had taken. Each setback in structuring a sense of personal agency had reenforced the underlying crippling conviction that it was not for him. Feeling defeated in his efforts, he had regularly fallen into a state of despondency and victimhood until, this having run its course, he was able tentatively to make another start. So he was prevented from pursuing many opportunities that might have lay open to him, and he was forced to abandon various pathways for which his gifts might have fit him.

As the analysis illuminated this underlying conflict, he was able to take certain steps that he had hitherto avoided. Consequently, he obtained a number of highly desirable commissions, and other promising professional doors also opened to him.

Mr. N began a session at this time by saying that he had a strange mixture of feelings. During the weekend he had begun to accelerate in his thinking and in his writing, he said, in a way that he had done ten years ago and not since then. However, he had again become depressed and could not get back to his work.

The analyst asked him if he was aware of what might have triggered the switch. He responded in a most familiar depressed tone of voice, "Every time I open the paper, I read about Tanglewood and Aspen. I read about all my old friends who are performing there. They've all been writing music, and naturally they're the ones who get invited," he said, sounding more and more lifeless. Once more he was being left out. "At my age" he went on as if in attempting to write he had been indulging himself in the most ridiculous of delusions," I feel totally invisible!" As the session continued, it developed that, in fact, his mood had shifted right after he first noticed the "acceleration" in the work and before he read the news report about his friend. "I was trying to get the work started and I felt I was dragging my feet", he recalled. "No career in the movies and nothing in serious music. Unemployed and unemployable. Nothing to show for all these years but frustration and disappointment and an empty life."

After some time I said, "As the work accelerates and you begin to feel enthusiastic, you feel something holding you back and once again automatically feel that that means it's not to be. Then your *depression* begins to accelerate, and that then threatens to bring your enthusiasm and your music to a full stop!"

Mr. N then recalled that when he had looked at the first results of what he had composed he thought it was very, very good. He stopped, paused, and then concluded hopelessly, "But what's the good of it. It's all for nothing!"

Mr. N rarely dared to express a favorable assessment of his work as he had just done. I noticed the progression of hope followed by repudiation and continued: "It seems that when you are pleased with yourself and have some hope for your future, as just now, it somehow doesn't feel right—and then it crumbles."

The session continued in this vein for some time, with me encouraging Mr. N to observe how a sense of himself as good and competent and having something to say in the session itself was constantly being submerged by another sense of himself as an inevitable failure, doomed to a life without distinction, and when that happened, everything in life, including his tie to me and the analysis itself felt meaningless. And I emphasized the importance of coming to understand this sequence, which recurred so regularly, as a shift in his state of mind, surely a disturbing matter, but limited and capable of being understood and altered.

After a time, Mr. N paused reflectively, then said, "What is happening to me is a little like Beethoven. He was going deaf and terribly depressed when he composed his second symphony, but he wrote that it was the sunniest and most beautiful of his works, filled with joy!" In 1952, Mr. N went on, he had played a recording of a concerto of his, and a well-known maestro remarked that embedded in its atonal elements was a basically optimistic, cheerful piece. The contrast between the relentless depression in this man's overt sense of self and the opposite mood he experienced in a sequestered corner that he could not sustain or elaborate in his life's work was becoming striking.

Mr. N continued, "Beethoven singlehandedly influenced Schubert, and Schubert was also a miserably depressed person, except in his music. And Mozart, terribly and incredibly depressed! I have seen the manuscript for his Adagio in B minor for the piano and it is filled with tearstains—there are dark blotches on it, but the first 15 or 16 bars is the most extraordinary music ever written." Here again appeared the cyclical lifting of his spirits, this time in an attempt to counter the sense of himself, reinforced by his recent illness, as weak and destined to failure, by aligning himself *through me*, I recognized, with the heroes of his childhood whose determination and gifts had enabled each to overcome the effects both of their physical disabilities and their own childhood traumas.

In the last few years, Mr. N confided, he had grown tired of heavy music, but he was now realizing that the more he lightened up in the music he created, the more fear he had, the more vulnerable he felt. I told him how aware I was that he entrusted me with the knowledge of the love of life that was locked within him, that I heard how he placed himself in the tradition of those who have fought successfully and at great odds against a brutalizing heritage and did not accept it as their lot in life. And I said, "I seem to hear a plea that I help you understand and overcome your fears and help you elevate yourself from the dismal world of your childhood to experience the *happiness* of developing and presenting what is best in you in your works with pride and enthusiasm, as you have just done here with me."

"Happiness was never supposed to be part of my life," Mr. N said with feeling. "My parents were so unhappy. My mother was always complaining. Nothing ever pleased her. I never recall seeing a smile on her face. My father had no aspirations at all. He came to this country and settled to be a clerk in his brother's grocery store. There was no love, no happiness, no committment."

"If I could only conceive of myself as a winner," Mr. N. said hopefully. "But I have this script imprinted on my mind. There is only embarrassment and humiliation in store for me. And," he continued, "unfortunately the facts bear me out!"

Once again there was the unmistakable sequence of hope and enthusiasm about a plan and a design of his own—and reactively the script of himself as doomed to failure and his resignation to this anticipated and inexorable fate. I pointed out the process that had just occurred. I emphasized that the facts only bore out this automatic, recurrent shift in his state of mind, an inability to sustain any happiness; they were not a revelation of a blueprint of the future, which had in fact not occurred. And I suggested that this must be microcosm of what must overwhelm him when he was by himself without having any means, as yet, for counteracting it, just as he had described at the start of the hour. Enthusiasm or determination arise and then succumb not to a relentless fate, but to some process of his mind that had become tyrannizing.

Now Mr. N revealed that he was starting to have fears of dying insolvent and ending up in the poorhouse. Many associations followed in which he recited ways in which he had failed. He was a loser, he insisted. Even though he had managed to get the commissions, this would fail too, he could just feel it! "When I think about it," Mr. N then said, "I am just exactly as my mother described me—fragile, weak, unfortunate, and incapable." The mantle of Mr. N's victimhood was now gathering its own momentum as he continued, "She felt I didn't have the strength to survive when I went out of the house. And when I would manage to leave I could not get interested in what I was doing, because I would see her frightened, unhappy face and I would have to go home. Sometimes she would open the window and scream 'Tommy, come home *now*'—it was so embarrassing, I hated her, but I felt so sorry for her." Later on, at the age of 16, Mr. N had a concert in Carnegie Hall. He had been convinced that his mother would appear, and scream at him for staying out and that he would be mortified. This fear kept recurring over and over again in his later life.

I noticed that Mr. N's mood had now become more despairing as the hour drew to a close until it seemed his own sense of himself was indistinguishable from what had been reflected back to him by his mother. For him apparently no Beethoven was available, as he was for Schubert, to pick him up and transport him to some higher purpose. As this function had been assigned to me, I wondered to him whether he had been having any thoughts about me during the session or as it was drawing to its close.

"Yes, I remember that I did," Mr. N responded. "I thought that eventually you will give up. The damage is too great. At my funeral you will be there and say 'Cluck! Cluck!' disappointed in me like everyone else has been."

When Mr. N returned the next day, his mood had evidently lifted. He reported that he had had an "interesting" dream. In the dream, he and his wife were in Scotland. They were staying in a hotel and, returning to their room, found that it had been stripped, that all their belongings had been stolen, and that the room was in a shambles. They were told that usually the police can find most of what was stolen but that in their case it was probably too late. The police had, however, located one box. It contained a telescope.

He left the police station and thought "Where could everything be, this whole bunch of clothes?" Then it occurred to him that there was a warehouse around the corner. He went there, and there were all their boxes, packed in a corner. They returned to their room and fixed it up as if it had not been broken into.

One association occurred immediately—to the telescope. "It enables you to see," said Mr. N, "things you ordinarily can't see. That's the analysis!" He said he thought that the dream was connected with the fact that since the day before he had been writing a good deal, that he felt hopeful that he had found himself. The whole dream seemed to me to reflect a most positive experience of the last session. The telescope seemed to convey that Mr. N had now acquired a tool of great promise.

Mr. N noted that the day before *he had no fears of going into his studio*. And he had written a good deal.

Still animatedly, Mr. N told of meeting with a composer friend and said how nice it was to exchange experiences with fellow musicians. He felt more of one piece.

He was getting flashes, he said then, about why he had married Jane, his first wife. In his discussion with his friend, it became clear that his friend had arranged everything around developing his career, whereas Mr. N married very shortly after leaving home and then was saddled with a responsibility for his wife and children that he never felt as his own. He realized that he had gotten married because he could not be alone. Mr. N was recognizing now how he had repeated his childhood experience at a crucial turning point in his musical career, surrendering himself to the goals of his wife and subverting his own for the sake of an illusory security.

"The dream about the things lost," Mr. N reflected "is just how I feel. I lost something indispensable at an early age, and I am now trying to find it piece by piece. It is all there, and I haven't found it." Although he had substained his optimism for a substantial part of the hour, there was beginning to be a change now, a negative cloud creeping in so familiarly.

"This morning," he said, "I had a strange fantasy. I thought of being in the Army. There was a withered old colonel who didn't like me. We had a private conversation, and the colonel got angry with me and took me to a court-martial."

"Perhaps," Mr. N went on, speaking directly to me, "you don't realize the extent of my damage. The best you can do is palliative. You are trying, but you don't realize how damaged I am. Something positive happens, but then I will wake up and it will have been a dream. Then the alarm clock will ring."

I suggested that he seemed to feel that my confidence in him and in our work must be based on his being someone other than who he was, on his having to follow my course, not his own as it emerges and evolves at its own pace. "And you are concerned," I said, "that, withered and old, I will be disappointed in you for not fulfilling my dreams for myself through you! So now the very tie with me that stimulates your hope is being absorbed into the automatic background script 'It's not for me!' As if this were also foretold and not a function of the same state of mind. That these fears appear between the two of us is surely frightening but at the same time," I said, "it opens the way to a better resolution."

A touch of hope then appeared in Mr. N's mood as he said that on that day he was planning to go out and buy a certain set of rare recordings. "Why can't I listen to music?" he mused, revealing the extent of the internal prohibition against pursuing his own interests. "It's amazing that I want to be a composer. Many people have given it up. But then I don't know what else I would be—and I have a lot of things I want to finish."

"There is a weight that keeps pulling me down," he went on sadly. "The storehouse dream echoes what I feel. There is a storehouse within me that I can see and hear. I need to dig it out so I can reclaim what is rightfully mine. I have talent, but I can't use it. When I started this piece I thought, 'What a great piece!' But the thought had only just taken shape when it was followed by another: 'You'll never carry it through!' "

Mr. N paused. "My father visited me at a recording session some years ago where I was conducting a ten-piece orchestra, and he turned to my wife and said, '*He* didn't really write *that!*' Parents don't kill; they just plant seeds inside of you that grow. Even if I should succeed, I will feel, 'That's not me—I'm just acting!' It won't be me. My childhood was a concentration camp. Survivors of concentration camps just try to make themselves invisible."

The work continued the next day as Mr. N reported still another dream. In it he was with Sam at the beach. It was a festive occassion, maybe Halloween. Sam gave him a bunch of colorful shirts, and he took them but then he couldn't find them. Sam said, "The Christians stole them!" Mr. N thought, "Born-again Christians." He identified Sam as an old friend and a superb musician, a versatile guy with great promise and a good teacher but one who had never made it. He was having all these dreams, Mr. N realized, because of the focus in analysis on recovering what had been stolen from him. All these years he hadn't realized that something had been stolen that was rightfully his, and now we were working to have it returned to him. Mr. N paused. "This analysis," he said, "is a lost-and-found department."

Born-again Christians are soul-less, he said. They have no understanding of creativity. They are dead—people from the wasteland in this country as Mr. N's parents were from the wastelands of Poland. That morning he had read the newspaper and gotten a headache—there were 46 executions in the South. "If the more intelligent people suddenly gave up and allowed these people to run things, this world would go down the tubes," said Mr. N. "We're not giving up, we're no giving up, don't worry," I said and Mr. N laughed. "It was impossible," he said, referring again to his childhood, "and I became like Sam, a person to be respected but invisible."

During the hour, Mr. N expressed his optimism about the prospects that were opening up to him. And once again, as it had so many times in the past, the optimism simply vanished as the hour drew to a close.

"I have the feeling," he said, "I'm biting off more than I can chew. I feel like I did as a kid when I began to write and illustrate a book on paleontology. I remember the mixture of enthusiasm and doom that it wouldn't come to pass. Anything good is just a fantasy, like my father used to say. It is incredible to remember that there was never any encouragement. He would just laugh. He would never understand."

Mr. N's dysphoria had returned when he came to see me the next day. He complained of insomnia and was anxious and depressed. He had written a little the previous day after his session, and it seemed pretty good to him. But today he felt as if he were just going through the motions. He didn't know if what he had written was any good at all, and even if it was, no one would pay attention to it. "I have things to do," he said, "and this is a nightmare!" He felt he was sinking backward, that his whole life was going down the tubes. Even when he was cheerful, he said, he was in the grip of an underlying melancholia. He had been struggling with it all his life. The day before, he had thought of burning all his possessions. I said almost nothing during the session, but I recognized clearly from Mr. N's description that the same feeling of dissynchrony when he was happy, as he had been the previous day, continued to haunt him just as it had when he was boy moving out into the world and pulled back by being reminded of his mother's unhappiness.

During the ensuing weeks Mr. N gradually became better able to articulate this curious internal state that confused him so much about who he was. He had revealed before that when he was cheerful he was unable to shake an underlying melancholia. Now he could detect and relate that even in the throes of the most painful depression "there is a feeling of enthusiasm somewhere inside of me, but it is muffled. I am carrying around a weight! I can't breathe. I feel like I am a prisoner in my own body! I hate this depression." Then he said reflectively, "It's a habit but there must be rewards. I don't have to fail! My immobility is a manifestation of an earlier contract with my parents. If I don't go out of the house but am depressed, my father doesn't keep deriding me for what I want to do with my life, and my mother isn't dying because I will get killed!"

Mr. N recovered his enthusiasm, so damaged by his illness, and its meanings after some time and once again began to make plans for his future. Significantly, a cluster of musical ideas were taking more definitive shape in his mind. As before, each period of feeling alive and hopeful was followed regularly by a reaction: "It's all a fake. I'll die before its finished!" However, the balance had shifted, and he remarked that he was "able to utilize what we have been doing and push ahead."

Another dream was enormously revealing. "I am going somewhere away from home, and then I try to go back and everything seems totally unfamiliar. There are dangerous things all around and dangerous people blocking my way, and there is some new construction going on. In trying to find my way back, I realize I am lost because I have departed from my accustomed route." Mr. N supplied the interpretation. He was feeling endangered because he was not taking his accustomed route of giving up, and that is why he was getting lost. Now he felt that he was on a tightrope almost halfway across, and wanted to run back because he would get to the point of no return and there would be nothing to hold him up.

"I am afraid that I will become so interested in what I am doing that I will never be able to come back! And I am afraid I was never told that to be afraid is normal." Here Mr. N was beginning to articulate the subjective experience of isolation and the anxieties of depersonalization that had hitherto always brought to an end his forays into a world, a life, and a self of his own.

Truth, the familiar platitude goes, is often stranger than fiction, but it is also surely sometimes more cruel. The work was proceeding, Mr. N becoming more and more encouraged in the process of self-reflection. This process and the hope it aroused were also repeatedly drawn into the underlying negative organizing principle as not being for him or as inevitably in some way leading to some personal failure. Nonetheless, he kept moving ahead. He now had developed four works that he considered major; one was well underway.

It happened then that Mr. N, by a twist of relentless fate, was once more struck down. He underwent a serious operation and was recovering when I visited him in the hospital. I had feared that he would surely be depressed from the all but irrefutable confirmation that something would always happen to show that he was not destined to have a life of his own. Instead, although in pain from the surgery, he was anxious to get going again. He had work to do, he said, and he was relieved that his life had been spared and that the outlook for his recovery was good.

This attitude persisted into his convalescence until he gradually became aware of a serious complication of the operation. Mr. N now slowly sank back into his depression. Nevertheless, he continued his sessions regularly as soon as he could get to my office.

The black mood seemed impenetrable. Mr. N would appear in disarray, with bedroom-slippered shuffling gait, face drawn, and with the posture of an old man. A dream he reported three months after his surgery conveyed accurately how he felt during this period.

In the dream, Mr. N had cancer. One of the doctors attending him said, "You have a terminal cancer." "Where is it?" Mr. N asked. "In the spine." "How long do I have to live?" "About a year," was the reply. "Will there be any pain?" he asked. "Well, you're feeling pain now, but you're getting used to it," said the doctor. Mr. N, crying, kept asking, "Is there any cure?" "No" was the answer. Another doctor said, "Wait a minute, there hasn't been a biopsy," but then he looked and said yes that indeed it was cancer. There was one way of treating it that would inflame the cancer, but it would give Mr N one additional year. In the dream he wondered whether he would have time to write his piece. He thought not, and there was relief but a terrible sadness.

In two years, Mr. N noted, he would have lived to be exactly as old as his father. It was impossible for Mr. N to believe he could get more out of life than his father.

Subsequently Mr. N gradually began to approach his desk again, but he would be overtaken by the most extreme exhaustion. Frequently he spoke of giving up, feeling dead, and was convinced that he was not going to make it. But he became aware that brief periods of hope would return and then disappear.

The process of analysis at this point deepened Mr. N's attachment to me as he was able openly to acknowledge that only my hope, and not any of his own, sustained him. Consequently, the work involved even greater attention to the impact of his sensitive awareness and subsequent processing of his experience of me. Thus, for example, weekend interruptions became for him more convincing evidence of my disappointment in him and my loss of confidence in myself, which Mr. N experienced subjectively as a loss of support for himself. Then he could not work, and there would be a renewed ascendancy of his victimhood or failure self.

However, the persistent reinstatement of the bond began once more to shift the balance. I found in this phase that particular attention had to be given to Mr. N's experiences of my tone of voice and changes in it, or silences and how Mr. N was patterning them. I made no special effort to alter his reponses, recognizing the greater importance of permitting Mr. N's experiences to emerge in their purest form. A shift was first signaled in a dream in which Mr. N and his wife had had a baby, cute little thing full of spit and piss. Mr. N reported concurrently that he felt "somewhat positive." Following this dream, the importance of the emphasis on the preceding transference analysis became clear through Mr. N's associations.

He had noticed that as he grew older, he said, that he was eating much faster than anyone else. When he was a child, he used to eat slowly and his father ridiculed and made fun of him. "Slow poke" was the way he was characterized about everything, and it was now how he thought about himself as a composer. "No wonder when I am going so slow I am wincing at what you are thinking," he said. Now it became clear that for Mr. N a most significant aspect of the terrible illness he had recently suffered was not the physical damage but his fear that it would have a disheartening effect on my belief in him and thus destroy his chance to complete his piece and his self.

I recalled then the dream of incurable cancer that he had reported after his physical collapse, and I realized more clearly what he had tried to communicate in the part in which the one doctor who had not confirmed the hopeless outlook had eventually caved in and given up.

This experience enabled me to crystallize an impression that had been growing upon me for some time. *The deepest source of depression in Mr. N, I became convinced, was the underlying belief that no tie could be formed and no pathway sustained in which the central strivings to give meaning to a life of his own and the disheartening internal obstacles he encountered could find empathic resonance and understanding so that he might ultimately prevail.* From this perspective, the loss of an object, so widely credited as the pathognomonic factor in melancholia, was for him merely an event that signaled the deeper loss of meaningful direction that had become engaged in a selfobject attachment that failed.

Several weeks later, some four months after being struck down, Mr. N reported the following dream:

> There was a Frankenstein monster. I understood him and knew he needed compassion. We were walking together, holding hands, and the monster started to sing an ode to the evening skies in the most beautiful tenor voice. I looked at him and thought, "What a creative, interesting man he is! That song could have been written by Schubert or Mahler." The monster was walking and talking. "Surprise!" he said, "Look who's walking!" The whole scene and especially the music brought tears to my eyes! I started to call someone who was coming towards us—X [a 20th century pioneering composer]! It couldn't be!"

Mr. N returned to the dream. "When the big monster sang about the night it was effortless, exquisite, like the most magnificent German tenor." Then he paused. "That monster was me," he said with a depth of feeling, and then, more softly and deliberately, "I have a song to sing!"

Another nodal dream occurred in this period. In it, Mr. N reported, he was driving in a car with a woman guide. They were driving over an enormous bridge on a smooth, wide, modern road—so wide Mr. N could not see over the sides. They were talking about Schoenberg, the composer. It was a comfortable ride.

Just before this in the dream, Mr. N recalled, he was leaving his house and not finding his way back, and he felt he was in dangerous territory in a slum area with his wife. It looked like Spanish Harlem, and they were trying to hail a cab. There were people looking out of windows. It looked like Dresden. They got to a thoroughfare that was lit, and all the taxis were taken. After that, he had the bridge dream.

His dreams were really a chronicle of his childhood fears, Mr. N realized. He felt the dream had been precipitated by his looking at his composition and thinking that what he had written was real good. He was pleased with himself and then got scared. Mr. N realized that the territory he found himself in was the picture of the world outside that had been painted for him by his mother. The tightrope wire of his fantasies, which he had to traverse to get from the world of his childhood to the world of music that had been foreclosed to him, was now, in this dream, a broad, wide, more secure passageway.

The final dream that I shall report occurred some weeks later. He was in his house. It was so full of people, partying, that he could barely make his way through it. He wanted to sell this house, but it was a wreck, a shambles that no one could possibly want to buy. He was conducting a potential buyer, someone he had known for a long time, on a tour through the house. They walked outside and saw that the whole roof had caved in and was lying on the ground, a pile of rubble. Mr. N thought, "Christ, I can't sell this house!" But the other man said, "It's really not as bad as it looks. You can fix this up, and it will be as good as new." And the man proceeded to show him: you take this and put it here, and this, if you turn it this way and put this alongside of it, and so forth!" Mr. N looked at him and said, "Really?" And the man said, "Surely."

They entered a room where little pieces of piano were broken and splintered. There were yellowing scores, ripped and torn, strewn all over, lying there, festering. It was like going to an old attic and seeing things that had been there 100 years! He felt repulsed, but the man said, "Look at this, you've done some remarkable things here!"

The dream, Mr. N said, was transparent. The room with the piano broken up and the manuscripts torn up was his whole life, in shambles and lying fallow. I evidently felt it could be salvaged—and I evidently knew more than he.

The house did have interesting arrangements of space, fascinating aspects to it, he was aware. That was his talent, but he had let it go into disrepair. Like the opening scene in the dream, he had filled this house, his life, with meaningless things. That's the way he regarded his life, as a leave of absence. Moving pictures, actors, directors, promoters have cluttered it up, just like the people in his dream. Mr. N paused. "It is really an elegant dream," he said.

Now he had a second chance, he mused. His opportunities wouldn't happen again. The dream was the picture of his broken dreams, and there we were like friends, no one screaming. I was just standing there, helping him look, not hurrying him and showing him how to begin to put it back together again piece by piece!

The process of sorting out, consolidating, firming up, and then elaborating his own authentic self-experience from various aspects superimposed on it has extended into an investigation of the creative process itself. Mr. N was able to go further and deeper into his own singular experience, to delineate and evolve more and more of what was the necessary, irrepressible, and, as nearly as possible, definitive utterance of this singularity (Rilke, 1963). The analytic process, here carried out from a stance of consistent empathic inquiry into the subjective world of the artist, far from interfering with creativity seemed to liberate it to find its own unfettered expression.

SUMMARY AND CONCLUSIONS

A history of a patient with a severe and seemingly intractable propensity for depression has been presented. Initially and for a long period of time, limitations in the understanding of the analyst and especially in his interpretive stance unwittingly contributed to delaying the unfolding of the story that lay behind this lifelong symptom. In two instances, this factor led inexorably in the direction of what has been described classically as a negative therapeutic reaction. (The account of the first of these, attributable to the use of certain traditional concepts to explain failures in life and in analysis as determined intrapsychically, has been described in detail in a previous paper [Brandchaft, 1983]. The second necessitated a revision of the traditional concept of analytic neutrality so that the analyst could grasp the selfobject tie that the patient was attempting to revive.) The analysis of these asynchronies led to a recognition that the tie needed was one in which the analyst could be experienced as a reliable, uncorruptible source of idealized strength, comfort, and conviction in support of Mr. N's efforts to understand his subjective world, break out of the closed system of helpless victimhood and death, and transform it to one of joyful creativity and life.

Once these obstacles had been removed, it became clear that the patient's depression was rooted in a relentless internal conflict centering on the meanings that self-differentiating processes had come to have for him.

Mahler, Pine, and Bergman (1975) have identified the core affects that organize and structuralize the evolving development of individualized selfhood, as well as those which characterize its derailment.

> The phase-specific, obligatory and dominant mood accompanying the processes of differentiation and individuation is one of unmistakable elation. And when this mood cannot sustain the individuating processes on which the unfettered future and creativity of the child depends, the dominant mood changes into soberness, then depression [p. 213].

The next stage in this process is necessarily the stage of despair to which Mr. N would regularly succumb.

Mr. N's development was interrupted at crucial phases in his childhood. Since he could not elicit the parental pride necessary to structuralize and vitalize his efforts to develop his creative gifts, his sense of self remained precarious and vulnerable to dissolution. In its place, a self-organization became structuralized around what was available in order to maintain a vitally needed maternal tie, a shared experience of hopelessness, despair, and victimhood. Mr. N's father responded to his son's efforts to escape'from the maternal bondage by repudiating his son's pleasure in the uniqueness of his gifts and beginning accomplishments; they were a threat to the father's own sense of self. Every attempt of Mr. N subsequently to follow his own trajectory was superceded by the claims of his parents on his incipient selfhood. And so the groundwork was laid for the intense, structuralized, intrapsychic conflict that was to torment Mr. N for almost a lifetime.

In the treatment situation when the analyst was able to focus on the patient's organizing experience and particularly to encourage the patient's self-reflective processes, a profoundly stable selfobject attachment developed. The important selfobject functions of the analyst included:

1) Attunement to and integration of the patient's relentless depression into a context of shared experience, if not of shared perspective.

2) Facilitating the emergence of and focus on the invariant underlying principle that led inexorably to depression—the automatic belief that he had to fail in the attempt to unfold "his innermost self."

3) Uncovering the developmental sources and origins of this organizing principle in preserving the essential ties to caretakers.

4) Identification of the basic conflict between the entrenched sense of self-as-failure-and-victim, an adaptation to the conditions that had been necessary to maintain his parental ties, and an insufficiently structuralized sense of unique and evolving self.

5) Attunement to the affect of enthusiasm, investigation of its ongoing fate, and the patient's need for the analyst to be its repository when the patient was repeatedly unable to sustain or recover his own so that gradually it can encompass progressively more differentiated and complex levels of experience.

Mr. N gradually recovered from the complication of his operation. He has completed a major work, and it is scheduled for spring performance. His song appears to have been given a voice.

REFERENCES

Atwood, G. & Stolorow, R. (1984), *Structures of Subjectivity*, Hillsdale, NJ: The Analytic Press.

Brandchaft, B. (1983), The negativism of the negative therapeutic reaction and the psychology of the self. In: *The Future of Psychoanalysis*, ed. A. Goldberg. New York: International Universities Press, pp. 327–366.

_____ (1986), Self and object differentiation. In: *Self and Object Constancy*, ed. R. F. Lax, S. Bach & J. A. Burland. New York: Guilford Press, pp. 153–177.

Kohut, H. (1977), *The Restoration of the Self*. New York: International Universities Press.

_____ (1982), Introspection, empathy and the semi-circle of mental health. *Internat. J. Psycho-Anal.*, 63; 395–408.

_____ (1984), *How Does Analysis Cure?* Chicago, IL: University of Chicago Press.

Mahler, M. S., Pine, F. & Bergman, A. (1975), *The Psychological Birth of the Human Infant*. New York: International Universities Press.

Rilke, R. M. (1963), *Letters to a Young Poet*. New York: Norton.

Stolorow, R., Brandchaft, B. & Atwood, G. (1988), *Psychoanalytic Treatment: An Intersubjective Approach*, Hillsdale, NJ: The Analytic Press.

Chapter 11

Reflections on Clinical Cases

OPTIMAL RESPONSIVENESS AND THE THEORY OF CURE
Anna Ornstein

The contributions of Drs. Brandschaft and Terman are clinically significant, as they both advance our thinking regarding those factors in a therapeutic dialogue that we consider to be potentially curative. I shall first discuss Dr. Terman's chapter. The questions he raises from a self-psychological perspective on the theory of cure are relevant to Dr. Brandschaft's clinical presentation.

Dr. Terman takes issue with Heinz Kohut for having retained the concept of "optimal frustration" as that condition which makes structuralization of the psyche—via transmuting internalization—possible. This, as is well known, Kohut retained both in relation to structure building as he conceptualized this during development as well as belatedly, during psychotherapy and psychoanalysis.

I agree with Dr. Terman that the concept of "optimal frustration" needed cleaning up, but I am afraid he did not go far enough in doing so. His argument, with which I am in full agreement, leaves ambiguities behind insofar as he could be understood as advocating the replacement of the concept of "optimal frustration" with that of "optimal gratification."

Shifting our theoretical frame of reference from conceptualizing psychological development as the gradual taming, sublimating, and neutralizing of the sexual and aggressive drives to a transactional frame of reference has consequences for our theorizing about what we may consider to be curative in the various forms of psychotherapy. In the transactional frame of reference, when this is applied to development, the formation of psychic structure is assumed to occur in the very experiencing of the transaction between caretaker and child. It is this developmental analogue, as it applies to the therapuetic process, that I shall subject to closer examination.

Bacal (1985) reexamined the concept of "optimal frustration" and recommended that from a self-psychological perspective the concept would have to be replaced by that of "optimal responsiveness." While optimal responsiveness is a useful concept, on the level of clinical theory it does not explain how such responsiveness can be thought of as curative.

To consider what may possibly be curative in a therapeutic process where the therapist strives to achieve optimal responsiveness, we have to question the usefulness not only of the concepts of optimal frustration and optimal gratification but what optimal means in a therapeutic dialogue (Ornstein and Ornstein, 1984). Is optimal to be understood as that response which exactly matches what the patient (or child) had subjectively experienced, a response that would "hit the nail on the head?" The question I am raising here is this: Is it this kind of responsiveness by the therapist or the repetition of a perfectly in-tune action by the caretaker that will, theoretically at least, account for the structure building that occurs in the course of psychoanalysis or in the course of development?

I am suggesting that in the transactional frame of reference, which is what Dr. Terman embraces, it may be better to think in terms of a spectrum of possible responses. What the therapist eventually chooses to say, how he says it—and importantly!—what meaning the patient attributes to what and how he said it will be neither optimal nor nonoptimal as long as it is nontraumatic. Rather, the response and how it is being experienced will be *characteristic* for this therapist/patient or caretaker/infant dyad and for no other.

Take the example of Eric. What if he, as a "bland baby," were not born to the mother that Stern (1985) describes but to one who was not capable of "adroitedly joining in and encourage, even intensify, the child's experiences so that he can move to a higher level of excitement . . ." (p. 193). Would Eric then be a not optimally but possibly traumatically frustrated child? Would we say that unless the mother responded to Eric the way *this* mother did, the mother would be less than perfectly empathic, that is, nonoptimal, in her response? I don't think so. Rather, we would think that Eric, with his unique temperament, intellectual and physical endowments, and the caretaker with hers, had to work toward some kind of a mutuality and reciprocity that eventually became "a fit" in which the child's progressive development was assured and the mother's own self was enhanced as well.

Infants pick up the caretaker's upper and lower thresholds of affect tolerance (Demos, 1984). Patients, too, "test" their therapist's tolerance for the intensity and nature of their affects and will unconsciously accommodate to the unspoken boundaries that are thereby being established between them.

Stern provides us with a spatial image where these crucial interactions between infant and caretaker take place and how they are mutually regulated. He says:

> Coping and defensive operations form in the small space between the upper threshold of the infant's stimulation tolerance and final crying. This space is the growing and testing ground of adaptive maneuvers and their performance becomes part of the lived experience of overstimulation. [p. 194].

I am suggesting that in a therapeutic dyad, optimal may be that response which facilitates a therapeutic dialogue, a dialogue during which the therapist gradually increases and deepens his or her understanding of the patient's subjective experiences and their genetic roots. However, no matter how empathic, accepting, and understanding an analyst may be, his or her personality and theoretical bias (similar to the caretaker's personality and unconscious expectations of the baby) will still codetermine the size of the "space" in which the patient will be able to develop adaptive "coping and defensive operations."

Note that Stern refers to overstimulation, as this occurs in an "average" responsive environment, a state that has to be distinguished from chronic and excessive overstimulation. The latter would have to be considered traumatic, resulting in the establishment of maladaptive modes of protecting the self from further retraumatization and possible fragmentation. These are defenses that interfere with progressive development of some aspects of the self and are responsible for the development of symptoms during childhood or in the patient's adult life.

Dr. Brandschaft's clinical example demonstrates that what we can so clearly and convincingly state in theory, or, retrospectively, in relation to our own case or the cases of others, is far more complicated and difficult to do when we are actually engaged in a treatment process. The case illustrates that to rekindle "the thwarted need to grow," that is to establish a selfobject transference or therapeutic "fit," is no easy task. What we expect from the infant, namely, the ability to elicit and to perceive our empathic responsiveness and to respond to it by a demonstrable forward move in development, is very difficult to remobilize in the adult patient. The reason for this is that what becomes reactivated in the transference is not only "the thwarted need to grow," but also the defensive measures (resistances) that the patient established in relation to traumatic degrees of frustration in the course of his or her development.

Kohut (1984), in his last book *How Does Analysis Cure?*, gave a detailed exposition of the self-psychological approach to defense—and resistance—analysis. He distinguished this from the traditional approach, in which defenses are associated with isolated mental functions that were governed by the pleasure principle and interfered with the analyst's efforts to make the unconscious conscious. In his view

> defense . . . activities [are] undertaken in the service of psychological survival, that is, as the patient's attempt to save at least that sector of his nuclear self, however small and precariously established it may be, that he has been able to construct and maintain despite serious insufficiencies in the development-enhancing matrix of the selfobject of childhood. [p. 115]

The implication of this view for interpretations of defense is that the analyst does not confront them and pays only fleeting attention to the details of the mental mechanisms involved. Instead, the analyst's attention is directed to the effort that the patient is now making to establish a growth-promoting selfobject transference with the analyst. It will be in this transference experience, different from the old "fit" in which the patient's self was severely compromised, that the possibility of a "new beginning" will emerge (Ornstein, 1974).

The self-pathology that Dr. Brandschaft described in this patient is very familiar to child psychiatrists. We are repeatedly impressed with the child's overwhelming need to be connected to and be accepted by an environment that is totally out of touch with the child's own emotional needs, and more often than not, this imperative need for connection with the life-sustaining "other" destroys the child's own selfhood and creativity.

The problem for the analyst, as I see it, is this: On one hand, he has to be able to convey his unconditional acceptance of the patient as he is, with his defenses and maladaptive compromise formations. In this case, Dr. Brandschaft did not question the patient's depressed, withdrawn, and at times paranoid attitude. However, along with the unconditional acceptance of the patient's despair, he had to be able to convey a sense of hope and the conviction that the patient was able to receive the analysts' understanding, to "hear" his empathic responsiveness. This is an extremely difficult position to maintain; the margin of error in how the analyst may be heard is very narrow. For example, should the analyst convey hope when the patient does not experience such an affect at that particular time, the patient can no longer feel unconditionally accepted. The patient's need to have his analyst enter and to remain within his severely depressed mental state made extraordinary demands on the analyst. It was important that Dr. Brandschaft accept the patient's guidance in this search for the growth-promoting "fit." Only when he could fully, without reservation, accept the patient's deeply felt despair could the patient move on to a different, more hopeful mental state.

The case demonstrates the limitations of the application of the developmental analogue to the therapeutic process; the limitation is specifically related to the fact that the developmental process does not have to take the presence of inhibitions, symptoms, and maladaptive character defenses into consideration.

On the other hand, I believe the developmental analogue can be extended to the therapeutic situation in another way. Should we consider, for example, that feeling understood and accepted as one is (depressed, withdrawn, and paranoid) may be equivalent to the child's feeling validated in who he or she is, we could then assume that feeling understood increases self-cohesion in a way that permits the gradual giving up of pathological defenses and compromise formations. When, in a therapeutic dialogue, optimal responsiveness creates the feeling of being accepted and understood, maladaptive defensive operations (resistances) may become unnecessary measures to protect the self. This permits the resumption of development at that point at which it originally became derailed.

In the case reviewed by Dr. Brandschaft, this process had to take along time primarily because of the patient's need to return repeatedly to a "safe position" where he felt maximally protected from retraumatization. Much of this therapeutic work seemed to have occurred on the level of understanding; explaining—the second part of the interpretive process—appears to have been frequently disruptive to the patient's effort to establish a selfobject transference; a therapeutic fit or space in which his creativity could blossom (Ornstein and Ornstein, 1985).

Dr. Terman has spelled out what it is, at least theoretically, that a therapist/patient pair has to accomplish in order for their encounter to have therapeutic benefits. Dr. Brandschaft has demonstrated how hard it is to achieve this "optimal" therapeutic position when the analyst's responses encounter severe vulnerabilities and their related defensive operations in a severely depressed patient. We are indebted to them both.

REFERENCES

Bacal, H. (1985), Optimal responsiveness and the therapeutic process. In: *Progress in Self Psychology*, Vol. 1, A. Goldberg, ed. New York: Guilford Press, pp. 202–227.

Demos, V. (1984): Empathy and affect, reflections on infant experiences. In: *Empathy II*, ed. J. Lichtenberg, M. Bornstein & D. Silver. Hillsdale, NJ: The Analytic Press.

Kohut, H. (1984), *How Does Analysis Cure?* Chicago, IL: University of Chicago Press.

Ornstein, A. (1974), The dread to repeat and the new beginning: A contribution to the psychoanalysis of the narcissistic personality disorders. *Annual of Psychoanalysis*, 2:231–248. New York: International Universities Press.

Ornstein, A. & Ornstein, P. (1984), *Empathy and the Therapeutic Dialogue*. The Lydia Rapoport Lecture 1984, published by the Smith School of Social Work.

_____ & _____ (1985), Clinical understanding and explaining: The empathic vantage point. *Progress in Self Psychology*, Vol. 1, ed. A. Goldberg. New York: Guilford Press, pp. 43–61.

Stern, D. (1985), *The Interpersonal World of the Infant*. New York: Basic Books.

OPTIMAL AFFECTIVE ENGAGEMENT: THE ANALYST'S ROLE IN THERAPY
Paul H. Tolpin

As I was reading Terman's thoughtful chapter, in which he takes issue with (1) the traditional psychoanalytic concept of the critical role of frustration as the motivating force in the formation of psychic structure and (2) the self psychological variant of that, namely that, to quote Kohut, "abiding functions [cannot] be acquired by the self without a preceding frustration, however tiny and/or fractionated from the side of the selfobject," I wondered how I could comment on a paper with which I had little basic disagreement. Of course, it is a fundamental question whether the major motivating force leading to the formation of "abiding functions," or, to use other words, whether the development of psychic structure depends essentially (the word "essentially" is critical here) on frustration or gratification—particularly in terms of psychoanalytic "cure." The answer to that question has far-reaching implications for psychoanalytic therapeutic technique. (I think that many of us would hesitate at what seems like a simplistic either/or formulation or one that reduces the motivating force in the formation of psychic structure to frustration or gratification alone; but that has been the traditional starting point for such discussions and it is therefore the necessary locus of ours.)

Terman divides his evidence into two groups. First, he presents data that has become available from developmental studies including those of Vygotsky, Kaye, and Stern. I shall not review them at this time except to note that they all strongly imply that the adequate responsiveness of caretakers rather than the absence of usual responsiveness (frustration, if you will) plays a dominant role in the formation of psychic structure. But I would like to mention a few relevant remarks developed from a discussion of these ideas with Marian Tolpin. Traditional theory gave little inherent reason for development to occur except for the effects of frustration. While it is true, of course, that there was implicitly an inbuilt, maturational tendency to move from one drive-structural level to another, the most reliable motivating force seemed to come from drive frustration. That is, the hallucinated wish for the breast, frustrated by a failure of gratification of the wish, necessitates a detour to reality to find satisfaction. As psychoanalytic theory changed, the concept of the facilitating environment influenced developmental theory more and more, although there were theoretical mixes that depended heavily on the earlier conceptualization of the role of frustration. While it is of course true that frustration is inevitable and inherent in the human condition, there are also ways to deal with it that do not depend entirely on the ministrations of the external world. These are the inbuilt mechanisms that are designed by way of effective signaling to elicit interventions and responses. In a sense, then, we are constructed from the start as independent centers of initiative, and therein lie important, effective paths for structure formation—that are relatively independent of the environment—though they must interdigitate with it. Thus, there are inherent tendencies that attempt to overcome loss or frustration and to reestablish self-cohesion. There is nothing we now know that favors the view that the child has to be coaxed into psychic development by loss. Rather there is greater evidence that the child delights in investments in the world outside himself and actively seeks it. Our responses to the child's search are crucial to his healthy development. Terman's position is bolstered by this developmental point of view.

The second body of evidence comes from Terman's own clinical experience. Terman has become increasingly convinced that "changes in [his] patients . . . occurred because of an understanding of the old and the creation of the new . . . [and they] arose from the experience in the analysis which had nothing to do with frustration." Further, that often "interpretation or understandings and/or aspects of the analytic relationship itself answered, that is, satisfied, deeply held needs . . . It was the satisfaction of the needs that opened new paths and remade old ones" (this volume, p. 114). "The essential question," Terman concludes, "is not so much [about] internalization but [about] creation. [Rather] the experienced response [of the responding other] itself makes the pattern. The formation of structure seems not to be a two-step process," (i.e., frustration of need followed by the substitute gratification, the bond of empathy) (this volume, p. 119).

To illustrate his ideas Terman uses material from *The Psychology of the Self: A Casebook* (Goldberg, 1978). He speaks about Mr. E. When the analyst stated that in effect he thought the patient was not psychotic, as he (the patient) thought the analyst thought he was, but rather that his feelings of bizarreness and his weekend of either hanging out in men's rooms or of remaining at home alone, painting chairs to distract himself, arose from this pervasive sense of loneliness, the patient burst into tears because he felt profoundly understood in a way that neither he nor anyone else had recognized before. Terman understood the meaning of the intervention to be as follows: "But what seemed most important to the patient was *the fact of being understood*. His inner state was accurately perceived and accepted. . . . By implicitly understanding the patient's need for the analyst and explicitly noting the loneliness, the analyst helped create an experience in which the patient did not feel alone or unattended" (p. 120, italics added). Terman's thesis follows: "I contend that the building of structure, the acquisition of pattern, occurred by virtue of the anlayst's reponse, [and] understanding; and the *internalization* of that new pattern followed from the experience of the understanding and was not created by the absence of understanding" (p. 120), that is not because of frustration. Rather, frustration only provides the occasion for the resumption of the experience of the responsive analyst. Empathic responsiveness then is the effective agent in the prolonged process of structure building despite the fact that gratification in the traditional (drive-oriented) psychoanalytic sense does not occur.

After citing Bacal's important 1985 paper on this subject and his introduction of the apt phrase "optimal responsiveness," to denote the motivating force in the formation of psychic structure, Terman, using his own terminology, concludes that it is the "dialogue of construction" that characterizes structure formation. By dialogue of construction, he means that we participate in an affective dialogue with patients and that by way of that essentially "gratifying," repeated dialogue (gratifying because it conveys intimate understanding, and implicitly, in-depth involvement) structure is formed.

As I said earlier, I find little to disagree with in Terman's paper. It is indeed my own impression from my analytic work that the positive intrapsychic connection between the patient and the analyst (based to varying degrees on the interplay between the transference and the content of the analyst's understanding and interpretations) is the major force in the renewed development and restructuralization of the patient's personality. This is not to imply that frustration does not play some role in the process, but I believe, as Terman has suggested, the major role of frustration is to act as the background stimulus for an understanding reengagement with the patient. Still, traditional analytic understanding and Kohut's (1984) insistence that "abiding functions [cannot] be acquired by the self without a preceding frustration, however tiny or fractionated . . . it may be" (p. 100) must still give us pause. It may be that structuralization is not achieved by one psychological method only. It may be that at different periods of development one or several psychological methods independently or in concert lead to the formation of "abiding functions." There may be different balances between interacting degress of frustration and gratification or types of each. Further, it may be that structuralization in adults in analysis may occur in a manner that is, to some degree, different from that which occurs in the life experiences of infancy and childhood.

Kohut (1979) discussed relevant issues in "The Two Analyses of Mr. Z." In commenting about Mr. Z's relationship with the idealized camp counselor who was understood in the second analysis to be "the yearned for figure of a strong fatherly man . . . ," Kohut argues that he "thought . . . that Mr. Z. would have obtained more lasting benefits from the friendship . . . if their closeness had remained free of sexual contacts" (p. 19). He elaborates this further in a footnote, where he questions whether he is still unduly influenced in his opinion about this by the classical theory of drive sublimation, that is, ". . . whether sexual activities between self and selfobject preclude structure formation . . ." (p. 19, n.4). He believes the issue is still in need of empirical investigation. He continues, "The most important structure building, occurs after all, in childhood, and it is not only not prevented by vigorous and sensually stimulating contact with the selfobjects . . . but seems to be enhanced by it." Also relevant to the general issue of structure formation is his discussion of Mr. Z's revelation of his childhood anal masturbatory activities, which included smelling and tasting his own feces. His shame at recalling these memories was overwhelmingly intense. Yet they "were well within tolerable limits because he had come to understand for the first time, *in empathic consonance with another human being* . . ." (p. 17, italics added), what these activities really meant.

In addition, there are Kohut's (unwritten) comments about the role of the understanding phase of the analysis. He often said that in many patients it constituted the most prolonged period of analytic work. Implicit in that, I believe, is a strong belief in the self-organizing value of just the kind of positive, affective participation with the patient that is a kind of "gratification"—nonlibidinal but strongly self-satisfying and self-enhancing.

Notwithstanding the preceding, I think, as I said earlier, that Terman's reasoning about this is persuasive; and while it does not rule out the critical, mobilizing role of frustration in the formation of structure, it does seem to me that the question boils down to what is the *indispensable* ingredient for the development of a healthy self-organization or for a successful *analytic* endeavor. And it seems to me that the optimal empathic engagement of the analyst and the patient are the crucial determinants of that.

Dr. Brandchaft's contribution is nothing if it is not inspirational—and it is certainly that, and more. Brandchaft chronicles the vicissitudes in the life and therapy of his hapless patient with sensitivity and warmth. At the same time, he maintains the objectivity of a seasoned analyst who attends as carefully to his own misunderstandings of his patient's dynamics as he does to the transference—clearly an excellent thing in a therapist.

It is Brandchaft's contention (borrowed from Atwood and Stolorow, 1984) that pathogenesis can be understood in terms of "severe dysjunctures or asynchronies" between the parents' and the child's idiosyncrasies of needs, feelings, states of mind ("subjectivities") in which the "primary developmental needs of the child" do not meet with an adequate response. When this occurs, the plastic psychological structure of the child accommodates to what is required by the adult. In other words, the child takes what it can get from the parents and conforms to the parents' attitudes and behavior, no matter how inimical they may ultimately be, in order to maintain his own psychological stability, which depends on them. One outcome of this may be symptoms in which archaic aspects of the self are maintained "in conflict with, or in isolation from, the unresponsive selfobjects." For Mr. N, Brandchaft's patient, this meant that his own inherent, "individualized vitality" had to be quashed in order to maintain "indispensable" selfobject ties to his parents. For Mr. N, this submissive solution led to a dominating depressive affect, the consequence of the continuing desire to grow and the continuing need for a tie to objects which was incompatible with that desire.

While I have some difficulty with the sufficiency of the preceding abstract for understanding Mr. N's profound depressive core, I do think that the notion that the child must bend his "self" to conform to his selfobject's characterology and pathology is a useful one. While the clinical material from which that formulation is derived does give an immediate sense of the stultifying effects of the parents' devastating attitudes that led to Mr. N's sense of inescapable valuelessness, it seems to me that the massiveness of this depressive reaction must have its origins in even earlier, or at least other, maternal deprivations. However, my question about the sufficiency of Brandchaft's theory does not essentially detract from his therapeutic abilities even if, in his mind, those theories gave birth to his understanding of and technical approach to Mr. N. And it is that approach which I believe is the significant contribution of his chapter.

After some years of limited therapeutic success from which the patient regularly relapsed, Brandchaft altered his therapeutic stance with the patient. His initial stance derived from more traditional psychoanalytic theory and clinical techniques that did not permit him to reach the patient where it really hurt. The ever-vulnerable patient felt as injured or depressed by Brandchaft's active or passive failures as he had been in his childhood. At some point, Brandchaft realized that to be effective he would have to revise "the traditional concept of analytic neutrality so that the analyst could grasp the selfobject ties that the patient was attempting to revive" (p. 152), this volume. That attachment came to be recognized as "one in which the analyst could be experienced as a reliable, uncorruptible source of idealized strength, comfort and conviction in support of Mr. N's efforts to understand his subjective world, break out of the closed system of helpless victimhood and death and transform it to one of joyful creativity and life" (p. 152, this volume).

There are a number of examples of Brandchaft's altered approach to the patient, whose self-regard was continually in a state of flux ranging from brief bursts of intense hope for extravagant success to collapse into states of profound despair that he would ever be able to make use of his musical abilities and that he was doomed to suffer the loss of hope for any pleasure or success in life. This "fate" had in the past operated as a quasi-masochistic but sustaining tie to his parents.

The patient had been depreciated by his father and infantilized by his mother. Nor could he expect any sustained attention or enthusiasm from either parent in any interest, project, or development of his own. In line with his new approach, Brandchaft was able to recognize the revival of some of these attitudes in the transference and was able in time to reconnect them to the past. He helped the patient to understand the now-structuralized need to retreat from the possibility of success to an indispensable tie to both internalized parents, a tie that took precedence over anything else. But he went beyond that, too. When in a better mood the patient spoke of his fervent devotion to and love for music and his identification with or idealization of psychologically afflicted greats in the history of music who had overcome their disabilities, Brandchaft told him how aware he was "that he entrusted me with the knowledge of the love of life that is locked within him" (p. 142, this volume). He said that he heard "a plea that I help you understand and overcome your fears and help you elevate yourself from your dismal world of your childhood to experience the *happiness* of developing and presenting what is best in you, in your works with pride and enthusiasm, as you have just done here with me" (p. 142). Later, when his attachment to the analyst was less problematic, Mr. N acknowledged that only his analyst's hope and not any of his own sustained him. Mr. N's sense that the analyst's advocacy of him and his persistent efforts to understand him were unflagging was illustrated in a dream in which the patient, with his wife, at first found himself in a dangerous slum or bombed out city, unable to find the way back home and unable to locate an available taxi. He then found himself in a car with a woman guide, driving over a bridge on a wide, modern roadway. "They were talking about Schoenberg, the composer. It was a comfortable ride" (p. 150, this volume).

In other words, after Mr. N had once again fallen prey to the embedded fears of an inimical, hostile, and dangerous childhood world, a shift took place when the analyst, as the woman guide who understood his essence, as exemplified in their discussion of Schoenberg, appeared. That confirming engagement with her enabled him to experience himself and the works in a quite different way, and he was then able to reinstate a sense of well-being and self-confidence as he drove across "an enormous bridge on a smooth, wide, modern road . . ." (p. 150). The previous "vitally needed maternal tie" of "the shared experience of hopelessness, despair, and victimhood" gradually gave way to the strengthened experience of the sense of the shared experience of the love of music. And the now reenforced sense of a recognition, acceptance, and encouragement of a core of self-pleasure and vitality, which had previously been too unattended to have a reliably viable life of its own, could now more regularly substitute for or offer an alternative to the negative tie to mother and father and the negative experience of himself as the doomed child. This development occurred as a consequence of the altered treatment situation in which a stable, selfobject attachment was experienced via the analysts' recognition of Mr. N's need for the experience of an optimally engaged, optimally responsive selfobject who could provide an analytic atmosphere that permitted the unfolding of his basic needs and a noncritical, even-valued judgment of them.

At the conclusion of this chapter (p. 152) Brandchaft lists five "self object functions" of the analyst that he believes lead to the flowering of the patient's previously stunted (arrested) developmental possibilities and the reduction of his recurrent depressive reactions. These functions can be broadly stated to be a fine-tuned empathic recognition of the patient's need for another's unswerving investment in him as someone with "a song to sing" (p. 150), that is, someone of recognized value who can expect reliably positive responses to his core self and who then accordingly does not have to remain a failed person in order to have selfobject sustenance.

Going beyond Brandchaft's five functions, however, I would like to add one more not specifically mentioned by him. Brandchaft states that "a profoundly stable selfobject attachment developed" (p. 153). I don't believe he will disagree with me and perhaps he was at least partially aware of that "function" (if it can be called that) which I believe plays a decisive role in at least the possibility of success in the treatment of such a profoundly injured patient as was Mr. N—and it probably plays an important role with other patients as well. What I think this additional therapeutic function Brandchaft provided Mr. N by way of his creative, ad hoc statements about the patient's inner life is a clear sense of *affective engagement* with him. That experienced quality arose from something within Brandchaft's personality, and it may be partially independent of what he formulated and interpreted to the patient. As I said, for some kinds of patients that capacity may be the most powerful force in the analytic endeavor. For such patients that quality of engagement may be the sine qua non for how analysis does help. For Mr. N I believe it was an adjunctive force that helped to revive the feeling that he could come to life again, that, indeed, he had a song to sing and someone who could be depended on to listen to it.

After all, we do have an emotional investment in our patients that is not simply countertransference in its more traditional, more restricted sense—with all its associated negative implications. Rather, I think there is something in us that makes our desire to understand and to help others not a neurotic problem but the expression of a highly developed capacity and an important part of our working psychic lives. And that quality experienced by the patient can have a profound effect. Further, I believe that the dual emphasis in self psychology on in-depth, empathic observation of others' idiosyncratic responses to their selfobjects and on self-psychological clinical theory as an experience-near theory strongly encourages the development and increased use of that valuable capacity of affective engagement with the patient—though it does not, of course, insure it. Brandchaft's work with Mr. N exemplifies the kind of personal engagement and investment in the patient that I have in mind. (Perhaps it might be considered the analyst counterpart to what Freud (1912) called the unobjectionable positive transference of the patient in relation to the analyst, but I would hesitate to link the two too closely, particularly since, in his written work, Freud did not expand that notion beyond a brief reference to it.) At any rate Brandchaft's becoming aware that Mr. N, who grew up drowning in denigration and derision, also nourished a sense of beauty that was locked in him, told him just that about himself in a candid and feeling way. And that rang true for the patient. Other things being equal, over time that kind of engaged understanding can be therapeutically powerful.

I realize that I may have opened a can of worms by raising the notion of the quality of the analyst's affective engagement at all. It spawns any number of important questions, such as its relevance in any psychoanalytic clinical-theoretical approach, the role of the patient's transference in experiencing such a capacity in the analyst, the investigation of this by the analyst with the patient, how much one should reveal to the patient about oneself, and so on. But an investigation of these relevant issues would require a chapter in its own right.

That aside, a case like Brandchaft's Mr. N is an invaluable resource; it reassures us that the successful treatment of an "intractable" depression is possible (and so may other "unanalyzable" cases) if the therapist can find the right intellectual scaffolding with which he broadly understands his patient and is then optimally able to use his own emotional resources to convey his understanding to the patient.

One last thought that embraces the subject matter of both chapters I have just discussed. From their own vantage points I believe that they have both addressed a similar issue, that is how does analysis work, and what makes it as effective as it can be. And as I see it both have concluded that optimal responsiveness, to use H. Bacal's term, or the "dialogue of construction which characterizes structure formation," to use Terman's phrase, or the affective attitude implicitly expressed in Brandchaft's paper are all related to the notion of optimal affective engagement which I suggest is an important and necessary ingredient in our therapeutic work with patients.

REFERENCES

Atwood, G. & Stolorow, R. (1984), *Structures of Subjectivity*. Hillsdale, NJ: The Analytic Press.

Freud, S. (1912), The dynamics of transference. *Standard Edition*, 12:97–108. London: Hogarth Press, 1958.

Goldberg A., ed. (1978), *The Psychology of the Self*. New York: International Universities Press.

Kohut, H. (1979), The two analyses of Mr. Z. *Internat. J. Psycho-Anal.*, 60:3–27.

_____ (1984), *How Does Analysis Cure?* Chicago, IL: University of Chicago Press.

PROBLEMS OF THERAPEUTIC ORIENTATION
Ernest S. Wolf

As self psychology moves from its revolutionary phase into that of a conventional science, it is clinical issues that hold our attention. The effectiveness of our clinical work increases as our discussions and refinements of the basic theoretical framework become more sophisticated. In this spirit I welcome the kind of conceptual clarification brought to self psychology by Brandchaft and by Terman in their respective chapters.

Brandchaft's case is a remarkably fitting illustration of the interaction of clinical experience with conceptual innovation that results in the fine-tuning of our therapeutic skills. He proposes—and I will use Kohut's terminology—that faulty interaction between the developing fragile self and improper selfobject responses from the caregiver may lead to conflict between, on one hand, the self's inherent need to organize itself into a distinct self and, on the other hand, the self's inherent need to be connected to a selfobject. This conflict, Brandchaft suggests in proposing a general theory of depression, becomes walled off, structuralized, and internalized together with associated affect states and, when the conflict cannot be resolved, leads to depression. However, one may question whether this specific conflicted child/parent configuration that Brandchaft postulates as the specific genetic precursor for depression is always so directly linked to the depressive syndrome. It is my impression that this conflict is one that really afflicts every self. It clearly is not a conflict of instinctual drives but one that is inevitably and inherently built into the constitution of every self. It represents the imperative need of every self to be a distinctive self while at the same time also it also represents the equally imperative need of every self to be connected to the selfobject in order to have the selfobject experiences necessary for survival. Everyone has had to struggle with this at times unpleasant aspect of the human condition, but not everyone suffers depressive illness. What causes depression in some and not in others is not answered by this basic human developmental vicissitude, though I grant that some passing mildly depressive episodes may well be an inescapable experience for all human beings. I think Brandchaft would agree—given the human condition of being thrown into this inescapable conflict—that it is the nature of the selfobject experience, which is a function of the selfobject's responsiveness, which determines whether there will be depression or not. Depending on the appropriateness of the selfobject's responses, we can talk about positive, that is, self-enhancing selfobject experiences and about negative, that is, faulty and self-diminishing selfobject experiences.

The case of Mr. N does indeed demonstrate this dynamic conflicted constellation, and indeed he manifested the depressive syndrome. However, it is useful to remember that depression, like anxiety, is also the final common pathway for many other, different types of dynamic constellations. Among these it is the absence of appropriate responses from the idealized selfobject that frequently are associated with depression. In Brandchaft's case, I wonder about the endless repetition of disappointment in the idealized selfobject parent of childhood or, during treatment, in the idealized selfobject analyst: disappointments that are followed by the patient's conviction of almost total worthlessness accompanying the repetitive disappointments in the idealized image. The unrelieved experience of incompetence becomes a self-fulfilling prophecy of actual incompetence. Why is that so?

In the analysis of this particular type of depression, the pathogenetic sequence can be diagramed somewhat like this: (1) The weakness and "unidealizability" of the needed idealizable selfobject is experienced as (2) a faulty selfobject response that causes (3) the regression, fragmentation, and emptiness of the self, which then results in (4) the experience and conviction of being bad and worthless. This in turn, leads to further (5) actual incompetence, thus corroborating the self-experience of worthlessness. The child cannot idealize a parent who is always fearful and unhappy. The child who develops without a reliable idealizable selfobject therefore will always have a weakness at the pole of ideals of its bipolar self. This weakness is experienced as a sense of badness and worthlessness and makes the child prone to depressions when during the course of life the ever unsatisfied yearning for idealized selfobjects is inevitably disappointed again.

The patient's repeated lamentations may also easily evoke in the analyst a depressing disappointment in himself and in his powers similar to that experienced by the patient and, much more importantly, similar to the patient's picture of the fearful and inadequate parent. The analyst thus repeats the childhood experience, in *actuality*, not just as transference, until the patient can recognize that the analyst, with his human failings, is indeed neither weak nor fearful nor depressed. And that may take some years, as it did in Brandchaft's case. The defect in the pole of ideals of the patient's self that is created by the selfobject failures in childhood, and that is subjectively experienced as depression, can be repaired only by a skillfully guided therapeutic disruption-restoration process. It is the total acceptance of the patient, including this painful self-experience—with matter-of-fact empathy, not with maudlin sympathy—by the analyst, without however, the analyst himself becoming a victim by sharing the patient's painful feelings, that allows the patient to have the therapeutically restorative experience of being optimally frustrated while being optimally responded to.

Which brings me then to Terman's chapter. Terman's chapter is a further step in the process to clarify Heinz Kohut's psychology of the self by eliminating from it the traces of pre-Kohutian concepts of structure formation. Terman is in agreement with and elaborates Bacal's suggestion that the notions of optimal frustration and optimal gratification can usefully be replaced by the concept of optimal responsiveness.

During the gestation of self psychology, Kohut gradually abandoned the drive concept as well as the strong emphasis on one-person, intrapsychic dynamics. Clinical experience forced him to recognize that the experience of the participation of another person is an absolutely essential ingredient in the formation or modification of psychological structure. He labeled the structure-forming process "transmuting internalization," and he retained the emphasis on optimal frustration as a precondition for structure formation.

Terman brings evidence to bear on the question of the necessity of frustration/gratification, and he concludes that only the satisfaction of selfobject needs, not their frustration or replacement, is the essential ingredient in structure formation. Both Kohut and Terman in their conceptualizations allow for both gratification and frustration, their difference being mainly a matter of emphasis: what is the major ingredient— gratification or frustration—in the structure forming process.

I submit that this may be a false dichotomy, since both frustration and gratification are indissolvably linked. As Bacal has stated explicitly, it is optimal responsiveness that is most effective in bringing about desirable changes. Optimal responsiveness, by definition, is tailored to the patients' need out of that specific mixture of gratification and frustration that will lead to structure formation in this particular patient. Furthermore, the designations "gratification" and "frustration" must be carefully considered from both the patient's and the therapist's point of view. "One man's meat is another man's poison." A cautious injunction by the therapist, for example, may be thought of by him as frustrating the patient while, in fact, this patient may experience this limit set by the therapist as a gratifying indication of the therapist's interest. And, vice versa, a therapist may believe he is responding optimally when acknowledging a patient's proud achievement while in fact the patient is experiencing this acknowledgment as a bitter frustration because it may sound matter-of-fact and lack the expected enthusiastic praise. In appraising the quality of responsiveness, the focus of the therapist's concern, therefore, must shift from general considerations, or from judging by his own needs and experiences, to the patient's experience as the touchstone.

Also, we have here a clash of theories. Terman's theory cannot be proved by his evidence anymore than the more traditional Kohutian theory can be proved. Both Brandchaft and Terman have touched on contemporary theoretical controversies. But it might be well to keep in mind that theories are neither true nor false. At least they cannot be proved to be true, and eventually almost all turn out to be "false," that is, not usefully applicable in increasing numbers of instances. Contemplating that sad situation may easily cause one to experience some not so optimal frustration and may lead one to attempt to overcome uncertainty and boost one's self-esteem by constructing ever fancier theories that are increasingly far removed from the problem at hand. Or, one might try to give up theory altogether and focus on the practical issues of clinical work. But that does not work either. Without concepts that give meaning to relationships, that is, theories, one cannot do any clinical work at all. Indeed, one cannot even gather the slightest scrap of clinical data without a theory to tell what is data and what is not. So, like it or not, we have to choose among theories, and for that we need criteria that allow us to judge which theory is best.

Fortunately, theories can be judged. They are best judged by comparing which theory is more useful or less useful for some specific purpose. Some theories can be useful in constructing a general psychology, let us say, while other theories might be more useful clinically in deciding what interpretation to make to a particular patient. I believe that most theoretical controversies in psychoanalysis arise from the different purposes that the theoreticians have in mind. These different purposes in turn arise from their different interests that represent their different personalities and philosophies. At bottom, most theoretical controversies are really clashes of personalities and philosophies.

These considerations can be applied to both Brandchaft's and Terman's reformulations of Kohut's theories. One needs to qualify each theory by stating its purpose. If one is greatly interested in constructing a general psychological theory that encompasses the vast field studied by analysts from Freud until the present day and in bringing the results of all these observations and speculations into harmony with the other sciences constructed by man, one will tend to arrive at broad conceptualizations like those of Freud. I believe Brandchaft's theory of depression and Terman's generalizations about frustration/gratification fall into this category also even though they address clinical problems.

On the other hand, if one is primarily interested in an individual patient and an individual self for the purpose of alleviating psychological suffering, one is best served by clinical theories that focus exclusively on inner experiences. By that I mean a focus on the singular, possibly unique subjectivity of a patient where clinically derived theories about the subjective experience of the mutual and reciprocal interaction of the analyst with the analysand are most relevant. In these clinical situations, theories about objectifiable and generalizable events—in contrast to subjective experiences—appear to be more peripheral and perhaps unnecessarily distracting from the therapeutic focus while adding little to the efficacy of the desired therapeutic interventions. The precise delineation of these two types of theories and their relation to each other may be more a philosophical than a psychoanalytic problem but would add greatly to a clarification of psychoanalytic theories.

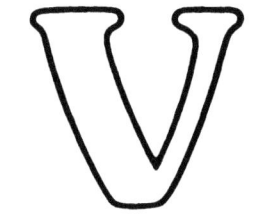

Applied
Psychoanalysis

Chapter 12

Arthur Miller's
Death of a Salesman:
Lessons for the Self
Psychologist

Howard S. Baker
Margaret N. Baker

A melody is heard, played upon a flute. It is small and fine, telling of grass and trees and the horizon. The curtain rises" (Miller, 1967a, p. 11).[1] So begins *Death of a Salesman*, Arthur Miller's play about Willy Loman and his family of failures. The play ends, as well, to the same plaintive sound. Willy Loman's father played the flute, took his family wandering across America, and earned a living by selling his handmade flutes. Before Willy was four, his father abandoned the family to make his fortune in Alaska. Willy's older brother, Ben, soon followed, leaving Willy behind, alone with his mother. These events help account for the tragic flaws in Willy's character, flaws that bring about his human failure and help create a family where the other members are also destined to become failures.

Death of a Salesman is a recognized literary masterpiece, but it can also serve as an extraordinary case study. In treating Miller's characters as if they were real people, we do not claim to explain the "meaning" of the play. To do so would rest on very risky assumptions (Holland, 1966). Our purpose is heuristic: The play can serve as an excellent device to teach basic principles of self psychology. All the "clinical" data is available for the student to examine. The interchanges are clear, and using video or audio tapes of the play gives direct access to human interaction and pathogenesis that is experience-near,

---

[1]All further references to the play refer to the Viking edition in the reference section.

intellectually accessible, and easily discussed and debated. A close examination of the characters demonstrates many points of clinical interest, and it is beyond the scope of any single chapter to discuss the multitude of issues presented in such rich literature. We shall concentrate on six areas that we find to have greatest saliency in teaching residents, graduate students, and colleagues: (1) the particular nature of certain human interactions that constitute failure in self-selfobject relationships; (2) any one person's ongoing selfobject needs may lead him either to meet or to fail to meet selfobject needs of another and, in so doing, to facilitate or even to overtly interfere with growth and structure building by the other; (3) certain selfobject failures may lead to the absence of intrapsychic structures that are necessary for vocational or academic success; (4) some aspects of selfobject failure may lead to suicide; (5) symptoms that appear to result entirely from unresolved oedipal conflicts may in fact be based on fundamental self-pathology; and (6) traditional conflict dynamics are intertwined with self-pathology in ways that prevent resolution of either set of difficulties. While considering these points, the reader can, of course, go to the "case material" (the play) for an independent examination of *all* the available "clinical" data.

The material helps demonstrate, in a clear way, that when the selfobject needs of one or more family members are exceptionally strident and difficult to meet, significant empathic ruptures occur throughout the family network. This system is likely to continue a locked-in pattern of interactions that may preclude the maintenance of a coherent and stable self in some or all family members. At the developmentally appropriate time, or belatedly, the parents and children may be unable to develop endopsychic structures that would enable them to: maintain self-esteem in the face of expectable failures, have sufficient drive and ambition to pursue interests and appropriately compete, enjoy creative and productive efforts that are an expression of the nuclear program of the self, calm the self, channel and regulate the drives, set meaningful goals that are possible to achieve, maintain a sense of connectedness with others, develop talents into usable skills, and so forth.

The play portrays people who are encumbered with significant structural deficit in each of these areas and who are, therefore, excessively dependent on others to fulfill selfobject functions. Because their intrapsychic deficits are so great, it is not possible for the Lomans to gain enough selfobject support to maintain satisfactory self-cohesion and vigor, let alone to belatedly reinstitute derailed development of self-structure. Their intrapsychic needs cannot be met through compensatory interpersonal solutions. Moreover, their unresolved oedipal conflicts create further resistances to the establishment of the intimacy necessary for effective self-selfobject relationships. For the Lomans, all these factors combined to create a witch's brew of conflict and deficit that yielded a father who was a failure and eventually committed suicide, two sons who were academic and vocational failures, and a mother who was lost in a quagmire of useless placating and denial.

In writing about *Death of a Salesman*, Miller (1967b) stated that he was trying to show us "the inside of a man's head" (p. 23). Thus, events in the play often follow a stream of consciousness, with sudden shifts between reality and hallucinations of Willy's past. In the following summary of the play, brackets enclose the hallucinations.

In the late evening or early morning, Willy, age 60, unexpectedly returns from a selling trip, exhausted, unable to control his car, and having sold nothing. His two children, Biff, age 34, and Happy, age 32, are home. Hap lives nearby, works as a marginally successful salesman in a large store, and has frequent, loveless sexual affairs. Biff has returned from the West, where he was working as a ranchhand. He was, in fact, a drifter and had been jailed for petty theft. He returns almost every spring, supposedly to settle down. Disagreements with his father impel him to leave after only brief stays.

Willy initiates numerous arguments with his 50-year-old wife, Linda. In their bedroom, the boys are awakened and discuss their father's deteriorating condition and how he upsets their mother. They lay grandiose plans for their joint success. (At the same time, Willy loses himself in a hallucinated fantasy about how great life was when Biff was a high school football star. Biff was the captain of the team and of Willy's psychic life. Although Biff occasionally stole things and was in serious academic trouble, these problems were ignored or even glorified because Biff was "well liked." Biff used his admirers and bluffed his teachers while his classmate Bernard was scoffed at for being too serious and scholarly.) A neighbor, Charley, Willy's only friend and Bernard's father, hears the commotion and comes over to calm Willy down. (Willy's older brother, Ben, appears to Willy, who showers Ben with admiration for his success in African diamond mines and Alaskan timber. Willy confesses to his brother that he is unsure of himself and of the way he raised his boys.) The scene shifts, and Linda and her sons are alone, discussing Willy's problems. She tells them she knows Willy is very upset and is contemplating suicide. Linda implores Biff to settle down and be good to his father. Willy comes in and starts an argument with Biff, accusing Biff of being a failure to spite him. Hap stops the argument by telling of their patently unrealistic plans for Biff to go to an old employer, Bill Oliver, to get backing for a business venture. Willy and Linda find the plan wonderful, are momentarily delighted, and retire to bed, relieved.

The next morning, in Act Two, Willy goes to his employer, Howard

Wheeler, to ask for work in New York, since he is no longer physically able to travel. Instead of reassignment, he is fired. He goes to
Charley's office to beg for money, as he has often had to do recently.
Charley's successful son, Bernard, is there; and Willy is obviously
jealous and wonders where he and Biff went wrong. Charley offers
Willy a job, which Willy contemptuously refuses. Willy then goes to
a restaurant where he and his sons were to celebrate his transfer and
Biff's new job. Biff has met with no success. Humiliated, he has stolen Oliver's fountain pen. He wants to tell his father that he loves him
but hates the life of a salesman. His father cannot hear Biff, and another
argument ensues. Willy goes to the men's room. (He lapses back to
the supposedly decisive moment in Biff's life. Biff flunked math,
preventing his high school graduation. He rushed to Boston where Willy was on a business trip, hoping his father could persuade the teacher
to pass him or perhaps just looking for reassurance. He entered his
father's room and, finding a half-clad woman, fled in despair.) Biff
leaves the restaurant, with Hap and the two women Hap has picked
up in hot pursuit. Abandoned by his sons, Willy is defeated and desperate. He leaves the restaurant, buys some garden seeds, and wanders
home to plant them. When the boys return home, Linda is wild with
fury because they walked out on Willy and because they consistently
disappoint him. She wants them to leave forever, fearing they will destroy Willy. Biff tells Willy why he finds peace in working as a ranchhand, why he can never be the monied urban success his father wants
him to be. Although not genuinely understanding what was said, Willy
at last feels and accepts his son's love. Willy has already decided to
commit suicide so Biff will have the insurance money to start in business. He does so, and a brief final scene takes place at his grave with
only the Loman family, Charley, and Bernard present. The crowd of
people Willy claimed as friends and admirers never appears.

These unhappy people have received surprisingly little examination
in the psychoanalytic literature. What has been written did not consider how the Lomans all seem to be encumbered with fundamental
self-psychopathology or how this prevents them from using one
another to meet essential selfobject needs. Concentration has been
primarily on oedipal competition and patricidal impulses (Schneider,
1967). The play provides data for this interpretation. Tolpin (1978) has
noted, however, that serious difficulties in the development of the narcissistic sector of the personality will preclude successful resolution of
oedipal challenges. Self-pathology will inevitably result in oedipal-*like*
symptoms that may obscure the fundamental etiology of the person's
difficulties, namely, developmental failure in forming basic endopsychic structures that maintain self-cohesion and vigor in the face of

stress. Careful analysis of the play clarifies Tolpin's point, showing that below the oedipal theme lies selfobject failure and self-pathology, that shortcomings in self-selfobject relationships have occurred over three generations, in the early development of Willy and his sons and in the ongoing family and environmental milieu. Students can observe how self psychology enriches family/systems approaches and how neo-traditional psychodynamics interdigitate with supraordinate self-pathology. In our teaching experience, these are crucial lessons. Particularly for residents and psychology doctoral students, not understanding these relationships often seems to create substantial resistances as they work to understand self psychology.

Writing before the development of self psychology, Schneider (1967) describes the second act as "sheer murder of a father by 'all his sons.'" Willy is:

> told by Biff [at their dinner meeting] that Biff has just compulsively stolen the fountain pen (genital) of a man who, Willy imagined, might have started Biff on his hoped-for rehabilitation. It is at this point that the father has to rush to the bathroom . . . in castration-panic; and the panic in the father is matched by the younger son's promotion of a date with two "babes." The meaning of this episode can hardly be missed. It is the ultimate act of father-murder; instead of the totem-feast in which the sons recognize the father's authority and sexual rights, there is no dinner. There is only abandonment. [p. 254]

The sons' actions may indeed reveal some unconscious patricidal or castration wish against father and father figures. All the items that Biff has stolen are obvious male symbols: lumber, a suit, balls (basket and foot) and the fountain pen. Happy specifically delights in deflowering other men's women, but he specifically chooses the women of men who he experiences as arrogantly humiliating.

The boys blatantly pathological behavior, however, will become "understandable only when . . . considered within the matrix of the empathic, partially empathic, or unempathic responses from the side of the selfobject aspects of the environment" (Kohut, 1977, p. 230). This intersubjective viewpoint sheds essential light on why a son might indulge in castrating behavior toward his father and authority males. Biff and Hap, in this view, have been burdened throughout life with being their father's primary archaic selfobject. Willy's need for constant affirmation from his sons (particularly Biff) has obfuscated their needs for a strong, dependable, responsive mirroring and idealized paternal selfobject. Consequently, they have not been able to develop sufficient endopsychic structures to maintain a cohesive self; so they remain ambivalently yolked to Willy, unrealistically hoping that he will eventually function in a way that will enable them to use their father as a selfobject. But, to have Willy function as a selfobject, the children must *first* function as their father's selfobject. If they could do that, then Willy might experience enough self-cohesion to be an adequate parent. They, however, cannot provide sufficient selfobject support for Willy, because Willy's needs are too great and because they (consciously or unconsciously) are enraged at a father who chronically demands something that they, as children, cannot provide. They cannot be Willy's flute-playing father who abandoned him. They cannot fill the boots of Willy's absent older brother, Ben.[2] They cannot be satisfied with the lives they have built by default rather than choice. Encumbered with narcissistic rage, to some extent, they prefer to get even with their father rather than help him.

Revenge and failure should not be understood then as merely a consequence of either sibling rivalry or the conflicted libidinal drives of the oedipal conflict. Those feelings are elicited by what is experienced as an unempathic environment. When Biff steals Oliver's pen, for example, he has been kept waiting for six hours. He wasn't given the courtesy of being told an interview would be impossible, and he is too desperate to see Oliver to realize that waiting six hours is absurd. When Oliver does leave, he does not recognize Biff and ignores him, forcing Biff to realize, "How did I ever get the idea I was a salesman there? . . . And, then he gave me one look and—I realized what a ridiculous lie my whole life has been . . . I was a shipping clerk" (p. 104).

Maintaining that lie is essential for Biff. Earlier that morning his mother reminded him that Willy is "only a little boat looking for a harbor . . . . Biff, you'll save his life. Thanks, darling" (p. 76). His father's psychological and physical life depend on Biff's doing something or being someone that is either impossible for him or very much in conflict with his own interests, with the nuclear program of his self. Fearing how he will feel if he fails, Biff tries to rescue Willy and is humiliated (castrated?) for his efforts. He must confront what he really was to Oliver, not what his father built him up to be. The helpless rage precipitated in such circumstances is so intense that for some it is disorganizing and must be repressed. It can, of course, present a serious resistance to the establishment of an effective selfobject transference.

Although revenge toward the father is obvious, there is but little

---

[2]Willy's pathology is intrapsychic. Consequently, environmental manipulation or self-sacrifice by the boys will not actually "cure." Most people with significant self-pathology cope with it, albeit marginally, through what might be considered transiently compensatory self-selfobject relationships. Family, friends, people at work, all are used to maintain a fragile, growthless stability. We suspect that under extraordinarily felicitous circumstances, a person could encounter such empathic self-selfobject relationships extratherapeutically that genuine belated structure building could occur.

data in the play itself that points *directly* to intensified competitiveness with the father for the mother's affections. Given the persistent self-selfobject failure in the family, however, we do not see how the oedipal period could be traversed without the boys' developing significant and persistent oedipal conflicts (Kohut, 1984). Seriously failed preoedipal self-selfobject relationships lead ineluctably to a developing self-structure too weak to traverse that period successfully, leaving the child with both fundamental underlying self-pathology and secondary oedipal pathology (Tolpin, 1978).

While both conflicted oedipal material and self-pathology are present and salient in the sons, if one of the boys were a patient, a therapist would have to make important tactical decisions regarding the timing of interpretations of oedipal transferences or of selfobject transferences (see Stolorow, 1986). This decision is important, since either set of interpretations risks disrupting the establishment of the other type of transference. For example, if drive-based oedipal/castration interpretations were offered to Biff or Happy when their experience-near feelings were that they were struggling valiantly to support Willy, the analyst might unintentionally "further reduce already vulnerable self-esteem and might drive a wedge through the therapeutic alliance" (Baker, 1987; see also Brandschaft, 1983; Terman; 1984/85.) These "patients" could well hear an oedipal interpretation as blame for libidinal attachment to their mother and for not being good-enough sons to their father. They would be likely to experience their analysts as claiming that their competitive and oedipally rivalrous motivation led them to want to destroy their father, whereas their own internal experience was that they felt little attachment to their mother and had tried desperately to meet their father's needs. While their rage is indeed real, it is both more accurate and more therapeutically efficacious to understand that its proximal cause is that they felt coerced to forgo the nuclear program of their own selves in a desperate attempt to bolster their father's self-cohesion. A complete therapeutic experience, however, would require examination of castration impulses, and these might prove to be derived from oedipal conflict as well as from the issues that we have already noted.

It is likely that, for the Loman boys, the analyst must first focus on resistances to establishing a functioning selfobject transference and then proceed to any oedipal issues that may be uncovered. Reversing that order would risk impairing the development of the all-important selfobject transferences, whereas proceeding in the recommended order does not normally impede the establishment of the object transferences—if the therapist is attuned to their potential presence. While this may be obvious to the experienced therapist, it is not to students. The material of the play and the student's personal responses to it can provide an excellent vehicle to illuminate this and other important technical principles.

Willy's unending and unmet selfobject needs are the central focus of the Loman family interactions. Struggling with serious defects in his self, which have their origins in childhood, and unable to recognize or accept responsibility for himself because of his endopsychic deficits, Willy must inappropriately use family and friends to meet selfobject objectives. They inevitably fail him, and he fails as a husband, father, friend, and employee. The nature of his dilemma is shown in a hallucinated interchange with his older brother, Ben. We are privy to a mild fragmentation and to frantic efforts to restore self-cohesion:

> WILLY, *longingly*: Can't you stay a few days? You're just what I need, Ben, because I—I have a fine position here, but I—well, Dad left when I was such a baby and I never had a chance to talk to him and I still feel—kind of temporary about myself . . . Ben, my boys—can't we talk? They'd go into the jaws of hell for me, see, but I—
>
> BEN: William, you're being first-rate with your boys. Outstanding, manly chaps!
>
> WILLY, *hanging on to his words*: Oh, Ben, that's good to hear! Because sometimes I'm afraid that I'm not teaching them the right kind of—Ben, how should I teach them?
>
> BEN: William, when I walked into the jungle I was seventeen. When I walked out I was twenty-one. And, by God, I was rich!
>
> WILLY: . . . was rich! That's just the spirit I want to imbue them with! To walk into a jungle! I was right! I was right! I was right! [p.52]

Although we cannot take this hallucinated interchange to represent exactly what "really" happened, it does show us how Willy experiences and organizes his life. And, as Stolorow and Lachmann (1984/85) and Wolf (1984) have pointed out, the intrapsychic organization of experience is what motivates human behavior. What we see is a man prone to fragmentation and without clear goals, one who needs the constant reassurance of others to give him direction and to maintain his self-esteem.

Willy's deficits began as a consequence of early self-selfobject disruptions. Direct disruptions occurred that led to traumatic deidealization of Willy's father and brother. Furthermore, their abandonment of the family must have effected Willy's mother in such a way that her ability to be sufficiently responsive to him was diminished. The play gives us no data about her; but clinical experience with other women under similar circumstances suggests that they are often overwhelmed and turn to their sons for selfobject sustenance in inappropriate ways. The son's legitimate empathic needs cannot be met, and satisfactory structure cannot develop. The son finds himself ambivalently enmeshed in an oedipal relationship that he finds both terrifying and gratifying. He hungers for a father or father substitute to provide direct selfobject supplies and to comfort and strengthen his mother. He cannot avoid, however, intense competitive feelings with that man. If a father or father substitute should appear, and if he is not understanding of the complex nature of the boy's feelings, the ambivalent hunger, fear of being overwhelmed, and competitive feelings will often destroy any potential for the needed self-selfobject relationship. One is reminded here of Mr. Z's dream of his father returning and bearing gifts (Kohut, 1979). In treatment, the analyst would, of course, be cast in the role of the returning father and must take great care not to interfere with the development of the needed selfobject transference. Again, oedipally based wishes to be rid of the returning father might also be present, but premature or excessive concentration on that aspect of the conflict might have the unwanted side effect of interfering with the unfolding of the selfobject transference.

A patient needing paternal attachment could superficially agree with oedipal conflict interpretations, leading the analysis on a prolonged detour that would accomplish little more than confirming the analyst's presuppositions. There could be, in other words, that most malignant form of resistance in which structural conflict *appears* to be examined while the weakened self is forced into ever more defensive isolation. The analysis would unwittingly function unintentionally to minimally gratify selfobject needs in the patient while never analyzing them. Although residents and other students are programmed to see the structural conflicts, the play helps to show how emphasizing them and failing to deal with self-pathology can lead to what is, in essence, an analysis of the "false self" (Winnicott, 1965).

The material in the play points to both oedipal and self-pathology that leaves Willy deeply entangled in ambivalent longings for male support. Because he lacks endopsychic structure, no interpersonal relationship is satisfying, genuine, or meaningful. Relationships cannot provide Willy with what he needs, or even with what he wants or believes he is entitled to. For example, when Ben told Willy that he had gotten rich in the jungle, Willy was so consumed with his need for anything from Ben that he did not even realize that nothing useful was revealed about how Ben's success occurred. Nor did Ben provide proof that the success was genuine.

Because Willy's needs for male support are so intense and so conflicted, he cannot find a way to meet them. He turns to Linda for both a normal and a compensatory self-selfobject relationship. He says, "You're my foundation and my support, Linda" (p. 18). Later he continues, "You're the best there is, Linda, you're a pal, you know that? On the road—on the road I want to grab you sometimes and just kiss the life outa you. [He is suddenly interrupted by a brief flashback to an affair he had with a woman when he was on the road, and then continues.] "Cause I get so lonely—especially when business is bad and there's nobody to talk to, I get the feeling that I'll never sell anything again. . ." (p. 38). He needs his wife to provide calming and soothing (idealizing) and to maintain his fragile self-esteem (mirroring). While this need is, of course, present in every one, it is the absoluteness of Willy's need that is problematic. If Linda is not present, Willy's internal experience is one of being intolerably temporary. Fragmenting, he must take emergency action to restore self-cohesion, and he attempts this through sexual stimulation. Healthier people, when away from home, remain coherent with readily available (although necessary) relationships with clients and other traveling salespeople, and, above all, with phone calls home. More mature selfobject needs must be met, but this can happen without resort to sexual promiscuity.

We understand these affairs primarily as sexualized attempts to obtain an absolutely required self-selfobject relationship or to stimulate a self that is depleted to a point of intolerable deadness. Undoubtedly, some would understand Willy's affairs as symbolic oedipal victories or as safe sources of sexual gratification (since his childhood oedipal victory leaves him feeling consumed by women who get too close). We would not be surprised if ongoing therapeutic material also confirmed the presence of these dynamics.

In any case, Willy is limited internally in his ability to turn to Linda. For reasons of her own, she is also unable to respond in a consistently satisfactory way. Sometimes she is helpful, but often she is not. Sometimes she can meet Willy's selfobject need, sometimes she cannot. Willy wants her to have good, solid Swiss cheese in the house. Linda, however, has gotten "a new kind of American-type [whipped] cheese" (p. 17). Wimp cheese! At the height of the family excitement over Biff's intended meeting with Oliver, Linda says to Willy, "Can you do anything about the shower? It drips" (p. 66). The repair was needed, but the timing deadening. When Willy considers taking Ben's offer of managing his Alaskan interests, Linda objects: "He's got a beautiful job here . . . . You're doing well enough, Willy! . . . Enough to be happy right here, right now . . . . Why must everybody conquer the world? You're well liked, and the boys love you . . ." (p. 85). Motivated by her own need for security, she cannot provide accurate, empathic understanding for Willy. When Linda tries to be supportive, her efforts are often based on denial, so they have little chance of success. When Willy confides, "You know, the trouble is, Linda, people don't seem to take to me," she replies, "Oh, don't be foolish" (p. 36). What Linda gives denies Willy's perceptions and dismisses his undoubtedly valid concern, thus providing almost no opportunity for the sort of forthrightness that is necessary for her to function as anything beyond the most fleeting selfobject in Willy's crumbling psyche.

Linda wants to be a good wife, but she just doesn't understand how to accomplish this goal. Her sense of self comes from her blind support of Willy, trying to manage household affairs, and attempting to make peace between Willy and Biff. What she is like apart from these roles, how she feels and thinks, and what she wants for herself remain a mystery to her.

Linda's inability to be genuinely available to Willy is among the reasons that compel him to turn ravenously to his sons for self-selfobject relationships. The play is replete with examples of how Willy needs his sons' adoration and that Biff is Willy's narcissistic extension—cheers from the son or cheers for the son temporarily maintain the father's self-esteem, grandiosity, and exhibitionism. For example, at the end of act one, Willy and Linda are in bed and reminiscing about the past, recalling Biff's big football game. Willy says, "When that team came out—he was the tallest, remember? . . . Like a young god. Hercules—something like that. And the sun, the sun all around him. Remember how he waved to me? Right up from the field, with the representatives of three colleges standing by? And the buyers I brought . . ." (p. 68).

Charley is another person who potentially could have helped Willy. Perhaps because his need is so desperate, Willy cannot tolerate the closeness Charley offers. He knows Willy needs money and an office job and offers him both. But Willy refuses the job and denies that Charley's advances of cash are in reality keeping Linda and him afloat. Willy avoids the supportive self-selfobject relationship that Charley's friendship might offer, just as patients resist the therapeutic relationship. For example, in the first act, when Charley comes over to calm Willy down, Willy brags about his skillful home repairs. Charley admires them as something he could never have done. "A man who can't handle tools is not a man," replies Willy. "You're disgusting" (p. 44).

Willy's need to hostilely ward off these attempts at friendship and help belies his fear and ambivalence and prevents him from experiencing affection from the men around him. His insistent and exhibitionistic display of "macho" prowess and his disparagement of Charley's masculinity say "I'm a man; you're not." That, of course, prevents the male-to-male twinship relatedness that is often necessary to preserve and consolidate male identity. Furthermore, if these needs are intense, they may (like other intense selfobject needs) become sexualized. When this happens, the yearnings are repressed and create an important resistance to the establishment of a self-selfobject relationship inside or outside the transference. While the play does not directly address the issue of homosexual conflicts in Willy, it raises enough question to provide useful teaching opportunities to examine how sexualized selfobject longings can terrify the patient and provide a resistance to the establishment of an effective therapeutic relationship.

Despite the intensity of his needs, apparently there was a time when Willy was successful at work, and that seemed to stabilize him. It was, however, the safely distant praise and hail-fellow-well-met attitude of the buyers, not his productivity, that affirmed him. Willy was hopelessly dependent on the responsiveness of the buyers; and when, in the inevitable progression of life, they retired or died and were no longer available to put in orders, Willy collapsed. The external props of others at work were destined to fail him.

Willy, then, is a man with serious defects in his ability to maintain a cohesive and coherent sense of self. Although he cannot entirely avoid the responsibility for his increasingly obvious inadequacy and failure, he must disavow this realization; and he is compelled to demand that family, friends, and job function as selfobjects. Expectedly, all fail him to some degree, partly because of their own legitimate needs or their shortcomings, and partly because of his ambivalent inability to accept what others do offer. More importantly, Willy is "failed" because his needs to obtain selfobjects are so developmentally archaic that they simply cannot be met in an adult environment.

Willy's suicide marks him as the most tragic failure in the family, but the other family members as well are terribly damaged by their interactions with him, particularly his two sons. Biff expresses his reaction to his father in an exchange at the restaurant. One of the women, Letta, says, "I gotta get up very early tomorrow. I got jury duty. I'm so excited! Were you fellows ever on a jury?" Biff replies, "No, but I been in front of them!" The women laugh, and then Biff adds, "This is my father" (p. 113–114). Biff has always felt on trial before his father.

The mirror that Willy provides for the boys careens wildly between grandiosity and humiliation, sometimes subtly, sometimes blatantly. When the boys are washing the car, Willy cannot help but give intrusive, unnecessary advice. "Don't leave the hubcaps, boys. Get the chamois to the hubcaps. Happy, use newspaper on the windows, it's the easiest thing" (p. 28). On the surface, this is merely a father's lively advice, but it communicates that they cannot wash a car on their own. At the same time that he sees them as incompetent, he offers this comparison: "[The boys are like] certain men [who] just don't get started till late in life. Like Thomas Edison, I think. Or B.F. Goodrich" (p. 28).

He gives Biff both false confidence and extensive, unnecessary, and contradictory advice about how to present himself to Oliver:

There's fifty men in the City of New York who'd stake [Biff] . . . . Don't wear sport jacket and slacks when you see Oliver . . . . A business suit, and talk as little as possible and don't crack any jokes . . . . Walk in very serious. You are not applying for a boy's job. Money is to pass. Be quiet, fine, and serious. Everybody likes a kidder, but nobody lends him money . . . . And don't say 'Gee' . . . . Don't be so modest . . . . Walk in with a big laugh. Don't look worried. Start off with a couple of your good stories to lighten things up. It's not what you say, it's how you say it— because personality always wins the day [p. 64, 65].

Rather than the occasional massive insults, which also exist, it is monologues like this, which imply incompetence and which occur repeatedly, that are the real stuff of selfobject failure. This peculiar advice is offered not for Biff's personal good, but in the hope of getting Biff to function as a mirroring and idealized selfobject for Willy.

Willy aggrandizes Biff in order to see the boy as ideal. The son becomes a narcissistic extension of the father, enabling Willy to bathe in the reflected glory of Biff's successes. When viewing Biff as the young "Hercules," not only does Willy fail to help temper Biff's grandiose, omnipotent self, he intensifies it. Biff's successes, furthermore, are not generated from an independent center of initiative. Instead, Biff's psychological job is dictated by Willy's need, so Biff must seek success in the way his father perceives success.

Because of Biff's expanded grandiosity, and because he cannot give expression to the core program of his nuclear self, he is often consumed with guilty rage that cannot be resolved within the unempathic self-selfobject climate of this father-son relationship. Narcissistic rage is then intensified even further by inevitable oedipal strivings and is repressed and given compromised and symbolic expression in the need to take revenge and defeat authority males as well as his father. By using himself as a club, by cutting himself down for spite, Biff gives expression to his rage, his guilt, and the defenses he concocted. Furthermore, when Biff is successful, those very successes might provoke envious and competitive feelings in Willy. They provide a comparison that directly reflects back to Willy his own inadequacies. Like the witch in *Snow White*, Willy attacks the mirror (Biff) that shows Willy's inadequacies. Biff damages his father if he succeeds or if he fails! The father is a mirror distorted in all directions—sometimes providing an unrealistically positive picture, sometimes providing a ruthlessly critical one.

While the play is filled with Willy's failures to meet his sons' mirroring needs, it is also gives abundant examples of failures in the idealizing pole. For example, when Willy finds that Biff has stolen a football from school, he half-heartedly tells Biff to return it. After Hap gives Biff an "I told you so," Willy changes course, saying, "Sure, he's gotta practice with a regulation ball, doesn't he? Coach'll probably congratulate you on your initiative!'' After legitimizing the theft, he reasons that it is okay ''because he likes you. If somebody else took that ball there'd be an uproar'' (p. 30). This theory seems to be central to all of Willy's thinking—what is important is how much you are liked. What you know or can do is relatively unimportant. Biff cannot use his father in the process of forming sensible, idealized, or even meaningful goals and values. Nor can a relationship with his father provide the impetus for turning talents into usable skills.

Because the father's need for the son is so great, the gradual, phase-appropriate ruptures in the selfobject ties between Biff and Willy do not seem to have occurred during Biff's childhood and adolescence. Biff was unable to establish relatively autonomous internal ambitions and goals. Consequently, a massive rupture occurred when Biff found his father with a woman sharing his hotel room. Without sufficient internal structure to deal with such an event, Biff underwent a traumatic, massive deidealization of his father and his father's ideals and values. Because both father and son were already limited by marginally effective internal structures to maintain self-cohesion, the event precipitated a catastrophic rupture in their mutual self-selfobject relationship from which neither could recover.

Preoccupation with Biff so consumed Willy that he virtually ignored Happy. Nor did Linda provide much for Happy, since she was so absorbed in attempting to maintain Willy's self-cohesion. The parents more or less forgot Happy, so the intensity of relationship necessary for a full selfobject tie was not possible between Happy and either parent.

Linda is a relatively shadowy figure in the play. We know nothing of her childhood. Apparently, she has little connection with the world at large. She works in the home and evidently has no relationships with anyone but her husband and sons. If there were neighborhood friends in the past, their homes are now replaced by anonymous apartment buildings. Linda is an isolated woman whose sense of self appears derived solely from her husband and her sons. Since her equilibrium depends on the appearance of the family's getting along and being successful, she cannot risk being authentic, direct, or confronting. Anything that would upset the superficial homeostasis must be denied or disavowed lest the minimally sustaining selfobject support she has be lost. She is left to manipulate the family matrix in order to maintain apparent stability. Consequently, she falsely reassures Willy and pressures her boys to shore up their father, while at the same time chiding them for not being successful and thus letting Willy down.

Linda's ideas about what is necessary for success in life are like Willy's, based on appearance rather than developed skills. Describing Biff as he left for Oliver's, she says, ''[He wore] his blue suit. He's so handsome in that suit. He could be a—anything in that suit" (p. 72).

One conversation between Linda and Biff would have an element of sardonic humor in it were it not so tragic. Biff calls her from Oliver's office, probably very much needing some calming and reassurance. What he gets is useless advice and intensification of the pressure he already feels. "Did Mr. Oliver see you? . . . Well, you just wait there then. And make a nice impression on him, darling. Just don't perspire too much before you see him. And have a nice time with Dad . . . Biff, you'll save his life" (p.76).

Both parents are unable to provide satisfactory self-selfobject relationships in all aspects of development, but can the wounded boys turn to each other? The answer is, somewhat. Happy's need to defend and deny his father's inadequacies, however, interferes with this relationship. Yet they realize that they need each other, and they do try. Biff says to Happy, "I'm tellin' you, kid, if you were with me I'd be happy out there . . . . Baby, together we'd stand up for one another, we'd have someone to trust" (p. 24). Perhaps it is his loyalty to his father, perhaps his interests are genuinely directed elsewhere, but Happy is unwilling to make that change. He replies and quickly shifts to his usual symptomatic solution of promiscuity, "The only thing is— what can you make out there? . . . . We'll be together yet, I swear. But take those two we had tonight. Now weren't they gorgeous creatures?" (p.24). He cannot risk change that would require him to forgo the narcissistic gratification he is able to get in his present circumstances, gratification that stabilizes his none to secure self structure.

Despite formidable obstacles, during the brief time of the play Biff appears to gain some insight and initiate some growth. He confronts his father:

And I never go anywhere because you blew me so full of hot air I could never stand taking orders from anybody! . . . I had to be boss big shot in two weeks, and I'm through with it! . . . I ran down eleven flights with a pen in my hand today. And suddenly I stopped . . . and I saw— the sky. I saw the things that I love in this world. The work and the food and time to sit and smoke. And I looked at the pen and said to myself, what the hell am I grabbing this for? Why am I trying to become what I don't want to be? What am I doing in an office, making a contemptuous, begging fool of myself, when all I want is out there, waiting for me the minute I say I know who I am! Why can't I say that, Willy? [Willy heatedly refuses to accept Biff's realistic view of himself; and Biff breaks down, sobbing, holding onto Willy.] Will you let me go, for Christ's sake? Will you take that phony dream and burn it before something happens? [p. 132, 133]

Willy is astonished. Although he seems to realize that Biff loves him, he is unable to use this belated awareness. Rather, he responds as usual to the affection and ignores the actual content of what Biff said. Unable to understand his son, he replies, "That boy—that boy is going to be magnificent!" (p. 133)

Confronting his own undeniable failure, and without Biff being the brilliant success he needs to sustain himself, Willy collapses from the depression of late middle life that Kohut (1977) has noted into irreversible despair and fragmentation. Death becomes preferable to a lonely, failed, barren life—especially if he believes his death will enable Biff to succeed. He thinks that the insurance money will offer Biff a chance to go into business. He says, "Can you imagine that magnificence with twenty thousand dollars in his pocket?" (p. 135). The suicide has a secondary gain. Willy hopes his death will make Biff successful; so the suicide would, in Willy's fantasy, reestablish the self-selfobject relationship between the two men. Here, suicide provides an escape from the unbearable pain of disintegration while simultaneously providing the illusion of repaired self-selfobject relationships and a restoration of the self. Frequent thoughts of suicidal patients, like "They'll wish they'd treated me better" and "They'll be so sad at my funeral," may serve a similar function of fantasized selfobject repair.

Willy can find no real life solutions. Biff, on the other hand, does appear to have changed. Even after his father's suicide, he comes to terms with both the good and the bad in his family; and he persists in his plan to return West and follow his own plan for his life. At his father's grave, he says:

> There were a lot of nice days. When he'd come home from a trip; or on Sundays, making the stoop; finishing the cellar; putting on the new porch; when he built the extra bathroom; and put up the garage. You know something, Charley, there's more of him in that front stoop than in all the sales he ever made . . . . He had the wrong dreams. All, all, wrong . . . . He never knew who he was . . . . Why don't you come with me, Happy? [p. 138]

Biff saw the empty depression that was an inevitable consequence of his father's pointless life. He experienced a traumatic deidealization of Willy's values and goals and fell into a prolonged collapse not unlike his father's depression. We frequently treat young adults who see the same absurdity in their parents' lives and are themselves depressed and profoundly unable to gain direction for their own lives. The problem of the Loman boys seems almost epidemic in the 1980s.

Unlike Biff, Happy has not been able to consolidate or clarify much over the course of the play. He continues to need to live his life for Willy and says, "I'm not licked that easily. I'm staying right in this city, and I'm gonna beat this racket! . . . The Loman Brothers!" Biff replies, "I know who I am, kid." But Happy continues, "All right, boy. I'm gonna show you and everybody else that Willy Loman did not die in vain. He had a good dream. It's the only dream you can have—to come out number-one man. He fought it out here, and this is where I'm gonna win it for him" (p. 138, 139). The goals and values remain Willy's; and Happy seems unaware that even if they were fine for Willy, which they were not, they are not necessarily right for him or Biff.

Over Willy's grave, Linda confesses that she has no grasp of what has happened to her family. She thinks that since their house is paid off, she and Willy could have been free. She just does not realize that Willy could not exist without Biff's fulfilling the essential selfobject functions we have described. Her failure to comprehend highlights that she was only marginally salient in her husband's psychic life. The tragedy is that Linda has so little awareness of how unimportant her defensive denial of reality made her—or how genuinely important she could have been if she had been more *honestly* available to her husband and sons. As matters stand, Willy left her in the lurch economically just as he had abandoned her emotionally. Her sons have provided little more.

The root cause of all this tragedy is not the lack of either love or the wish to be a good parent. Willy says to his brother, "Oh, Ben, how do we get back to all the great times? Used to be so full of light, and comradeship, and sleigh-riding in winter . . . . Why, why can't I give him something and not have him hate me?" (p.127). The answer is clear: basic personality deficits in all the family members.

The Lomans in *Death of a Salesman* are, indeed, a tragic family. But, they can clarify many important self-psychological principles. The family's members are prevented from offering each other the assistance they would like to give and all desperately need. They fail in ways that are major and in others that are quite minor, but constantly repeated.

They set conflicted goals and shatter each other's fragile self-esteem. Their symptomatology is overdetermined intrapsychically and by childhood and ongoing interpersonal failings. All this is done, not for lack of love, but because of overwhelming weaknesses in the basic structures of their personalities. We paraphrase Kohut in noting that it is not what they did but who they were that created failure and suicide and prevented resolution of their problems.

REFERENCES

Baker, H. (1987), Underachievement and failure in college: The interaction between intrapsychic and interpersonal factors from the perspective of self psychology. *Adoles. Psychiat.*, 14: 441–460.

Brandschaft, B. (1983), The negativism of the negative therapeutic reaction and the psychology of the self. In: *The Future of Psychoanalysis*, ed. A. Goldberg. New York: International Universities Press.

Holland, N. (1966), *Psychoanalysis and Shakespeare*. New York: MacGraw–Hill.

Kohut, H. (1977), *The Restoration of the Self*. New York: International Universities Press.

_____ (1979), The Two analyses of Mr. Z. *Internat. J. Psycho-Anal.*, 60:3–27.

_____ (1984), *How Does Analysis Cure?* Chicago: University of Chicago Press.

Miller, A. (1967a), *Death of a Salesman*. New York: Viking Press.

_____ (1967b), Introduction. In A. Miller, *Collected Plays*. New York: Viking Press.

Schneider, D. (1967), Play of dreams. In A. Miller, *Death of a Salesman*. New York: Viking Press, pp. 250–258.

Stolorow, R. (1986), Beyond Dogma in Psychoanalysis. In: *Progress in Self Psychology, Vol. 2*, ed. A. Goldberg. New York: Guilford, pp. 41–49.

Stolorow, R. & Lachmann, F. (1984/5), Transference: The future of an illusion. *The Annual of Psychoanalysis*, 12/13:19-38. New York: International Universities Press.

Terman, D. (1984/85), The self and the Oedipus complex. *The Annual of Psychoanalysis*, 12/13:87-104. New York: International Universities Press.

Tolpin, M. (1978), Self-objects and oedipal objects: A crucial developmental distinction. *The Psychoanalytic Study of the Child*, 43:167-184. New Haven, CT: Yale University Press.

Winnicott, D. (1965), *The Maturational Process and the Facilitating Environment*. New York: International Universities Press.

Wolf, E. (1984). Discrepancies between the analysand and the analyst in experiencing the analysis. Presented to the Eighth Annual Conference on the Psychology of the Self. New York, N.Y.

Chapter 13

Selfobject Theory and the Artistic Process

Carl T. Rotenberg

In preparing this chapter, I reflected on what had caused me to examine the interrelationship between psychoanalysis and artistic expression. My thoughts drifted back to my psychiatric residency, when, for reasons not then understood, I began to spend spare time viewing art in galleries and museums. I did not then associate this increasingly absorbing hobby with my professional goals, the acquisition of psychiatric and psychotherapeutic expertise. However, in retrospect, this connection is evident when I recall that one of my favorite paintings at that time, one that still repays my visits with sustained interest, was Picasso's 1932 work, "Girl Before a Mirror" (Fig. 1).

In retrospect, I see that there was an interplay between the needs of my evolving psychotherapeutic self and the formal properties of that Cubist work, which demonstrates the usefulness of fragmenting a unitary view of an object so that its different facets can be more fully understood when viewed simultaneously from different perspectives. The formal assumptions of Cubism invited an analytic fragmentation of an object into crystallised shapes and subsequent resynthesis through the viewer's reformulation, an activity that in retrospect I regard as similar to my apprentice activity in the clinical setting. Picasso's artistic success buttressed my uncertain professional self and aided me in the cultivation of a dissecting and analyzing professional self. All of this was unconscious, except for conscious feelings of awakening excite-

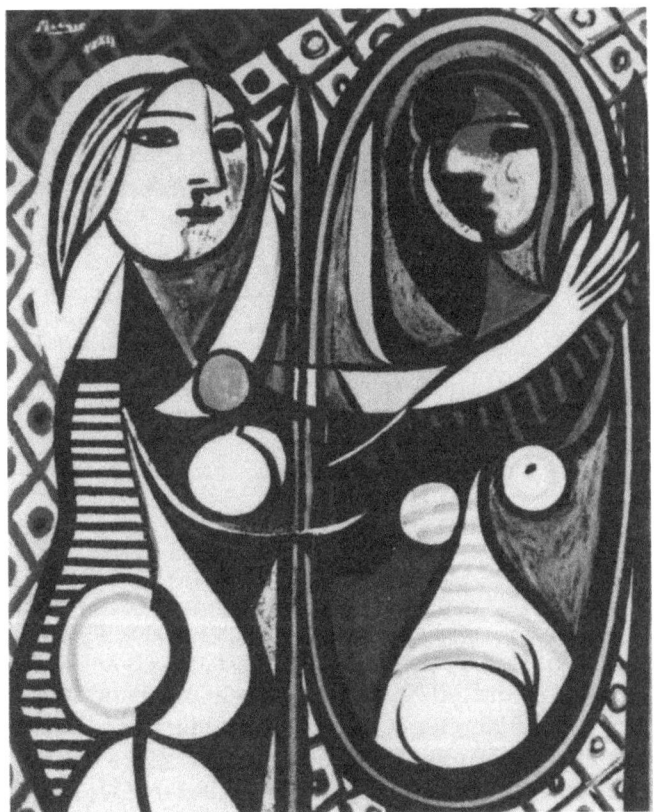

FIGURE 1.   Pablo Picasso: "Girl Before a Mirror" 1932. Oil on canvas,
63¾" x 51¼". The Museum of Modern Art, New York. Gift of Mrs. Si-
mon Guggenheim.

ment and the dimly palpable view that my education in plastic values
was not only pleasurable but served to mould my values more broadly in a then unformulated way.

   While Picasso's painting induced in me a thrilling state of absorption, I might, in other states of mind, resist those aspects of the painting I have described. Instead, I might attune to those elements which
communicated a feeling of immutable structure in the midst of change,
such as the structural balance depicted through assymetrical arrange-
ment of orbital solids across a vertical axis. In this vein, breasts, mir-
rors, and other ovoid shapes were offset reinforcingly against each
other. Alternatively, in a state of absorption with wholly abstract works
in the same museum (such as the canvases of Rothko, Pollock, or Hof-

mann), I might regret Picasso's conservative insistence on the reality of the natural image. I might be impatient with the conservative aspects of art work as a mirror of the so-called real world.

In fact, the Picasso work might induce a state of irritation and ennui. I observed that the artistic value of this work lay in the way its condensed messages could evoke differing states of self-organization at different times; and that to explain the psychological effect of this work, I had to look both at the nature of the work itself and at the way it functioned in relationship to my particular subjective psychological state at a given time.[1]

The dynamic psychological effects of artistic experience seem always to lie in a shared experiential space between the subjective psychological reality of the viewer at a given time and the artistic personality of the work's creator, as enacted in that particular painting. This space is similar to what has been designated as "the intersubjective space" (Brandchaft and Stolorow, 1983).

I have come to appreciate the powerful organizing influence that visual arts have for the self. Usually, when recalling specific art works that have moved them deeply, people will describe the subject matter rather than the formal content, and they will express considerable frustration when asked to account for the formal reasons they were affected by a specific art work as opposed to one of a similar subject by another artist (e.g., Why is this landscape so moving rather than another?). Discussion of the formal properties of a work can produce discomfort, followed by the viewer's abashed assertion of an inability to express or even consciously perceive formal influences. Response to formal innovation is both compelling and frustrating. It is remarkable, in this connection, how people return to galleries in throngs to view works they consciously repudiate with scornful laughter and judgments like "That's not art!" This interaction is evidence of the interplay of insight and resistance, and it suggests the organizing influences of art work on self-experience.

I have come to realize from patients, from written descriptions in the literature, from artists, and from my own subjective experiences that to participate in a visual work's aesthetic meaning is not only pleasurable, but, more to the point, transforms the participating, viewing self. In different ways, this is true whether or not the self in relation to the art work is that of its creator or of a member of its intended au-

---

[1]I am reminded of Freud's (1914) fascination with Michelangelo's Moses. In his paper, one notes his ambitendency in relation to that art work and the feedback loop between the particular work of art and Freud's set of needs, perceptions, and responses to the work at a given time. His paper depicted Freud's intellectual and creative struggles as he interacted dialectically with the 'Moses' sculpture.

dience. In a complex interaction, artists establish an interplay between the communicative aspects of their own work and their ambitiousness of development, seeking to reach ever-greater heights of artistic accomplishment. The perceived potentially organizing effects of a work are not an isolated or permanent property of the work's content; they interact with the self-state of the viewer at a given instant.

Similarly, in artists' accounts of their experiences while creating (both oral accounts and in the literature), they described a certain interaction between their creative working self and the "personality" of the work as they experienced it evolving at a given moment. They described an expressive process, unconsciously shaped and experienced as spontaneous and uncontrived, in which the particular details of an unfinished work would somehow speak to them and convey what their next steps should be.

There is a particular quality of interplay between the organizing properties (or *disorganizing* properties) of the work and the *creative* self of the person who is working. (With regard to disorganizing properties, see Kohut, 1976; and Ehrenzweig, 1967.) Even the first mark on the surface of the canvas already has some informing and organizing potential for the subsequent interventions of the artist as he works.[2] Another significant aspect of the self-experience of the artist is the "deep inner necessity" described by Kandinsky (1912), which illustrates the felt absolute requirement, a kind of drivenness, to continue working on the further evolution of his aesthetic knowledge, skill, and style and to devote his whole life to that priority.

Psychoanalyis, the science of complex human psychological states, should take the full dimensionality of the artistic experience into account, including the transformational potentialities of art for the self. Discussion of the artistic process in the light of newer psychoanalytic concepts is relevant, since more classical notions have taken us only so far in understanding it. (Kris, 1952; Ehrenzweig, 1967; Rose, 1980). The unique art object, which in this discussion is limited to the visual arts of painting and drawing (although the ideas may apply in other artistic areas), is a mediating link between the psychological subjectivities of artist and viewer.

This chapter's broader clinical relevance is that creativity is a major transformational force in the life of everyone. I shall examine the heuris-

---

[2]It is this aspect of interplay which led Picasso to comment, "A picture is not thought out and settled beforehand. While it is being done it changes as one's thoughts change. And when it is finished, it still goes on changing, according to the state of mind of whoever is looking at it. A picture lives a life like a living creature, undergoing the changes imposed on us by our life from day to day. This is natural enough, as the picture lives only through the man who is looking at it" (Picasso, in Barr, 1946, p. 272).

tic usefulness of the selfobject concept in the study of the artistic process. The implications of seeing the art object as "true" object have been reviewed elsewhere (Weissman, 1971) The focus here is on how the art object may be experienced as selfobject. I have reviewed some of the implications of this elsewhere. (Rotenberg, 1984–1985) The view of the self being discussed here stresses a cohesive structuring of goals and values into potentials for action, with the aim of self-realization. The self it delineates is a "supraordinate self," that is, a supraordinate configuration whose significance transcends that of the sum of its parts" (Kohut, 1977, p. 97). The personality as a whole, or the self in its essence, is most fruitfully understood "as a hierarchy of potentials for actions, i.e, a of of both organismic and subjective goals as modified by a system of values" (Gedo, 1979; see also Basch, 1975; Bruner, 1984)

We use the term "selfobject" to refer to an object *experienced subjectively* as serving selfobject functions. This definition is appropriate for an object, albeit an inanimate one, that contains within it many interweaving and variegated levels of meaning and areas for interpretations, such as the art object. It suggests that an important dimension of the aesthetic experience ripe for exploration is the various functions that the art object can serve both for the one who creates it and the one who participates in this creation through vicarious introspection. This stress on functions is offered tentatively, since, while self psychology stresses the functioning of the selfobject for the self, it nevertheless has so far adumbrated only rather generalized categories of functioning. Kohut (1983) assigned the further depiction of the nature of selfobject functioning as a research goal for self psychology. Possibilities for further research in this area are suggested by the subtle processes witnessed in the creation and appreciation of art. Here psychoanalysis has possibilities of joining its insights with those of perceptual psychology, so that the process of the communication of values, their transmission, and their subsequent internalization into the self, together with their accompanying affects, can be more completely understood and clearly delineated. Two of these affects, the experience of the sublime and the sense of inspiration, are particularly characteristic of the creative process.

When we encounter a new painting, we are forced by the actively prehensile quality of our perceptions to react to it and interpret it, if only for a second. Each one of us will react differently. Some might turn away, relatively uninterested, thinking something like, "What on earth is that?" Others will seek more prolonged engagement. The first reaction to a work does not necessarily predict its eventual significance. In fact, it frequently happens that spectators will enjoy a meaningful and lasting relationship to a work they initially found unattractive. With any painting, each of us will employ our own recipe of artistic "empathy" (Oremland, 1984) with the work's subject matter and formal contents. To the extent that we resonate with it, we will lose our sense of separation from it as an object, and our self-experience will begin to become congruent with it. Our connectedness with a work will depend on the work's quality and on the self-state and set of needs with which we approach it. We abandon a sense of separateness with the art object to establish a momentary fusion with it, a transient coextensiveness (Rotenberg, 1984), a suffusing (Milner, 1957), a blending, along with an accompanying temporary loss of self. Berenson (1950) has described the aesthetic moment as "that flitting instant, so brief as to be almost timeless, when the spectator is at one with the work of art . . ." (p. 80). This is not an unregulated loss of boundaries, which would suggest merger of a pathological degree. Rather, it is selective, optative, delegated, and reversible at will, even though the temporary fusion can be intense and ascend to feelings of the sublime.

To understand an art work's capacity to affect the self, we have to examine its contents, the qualities of form and composition that give it meaning. Let us illustrate this by examining a particular painting, "A Sunday Afternoon in the Island of La Grand Jatte" (Fig. 2). This famous painting was painted a century ago. Keeping in mind the art-

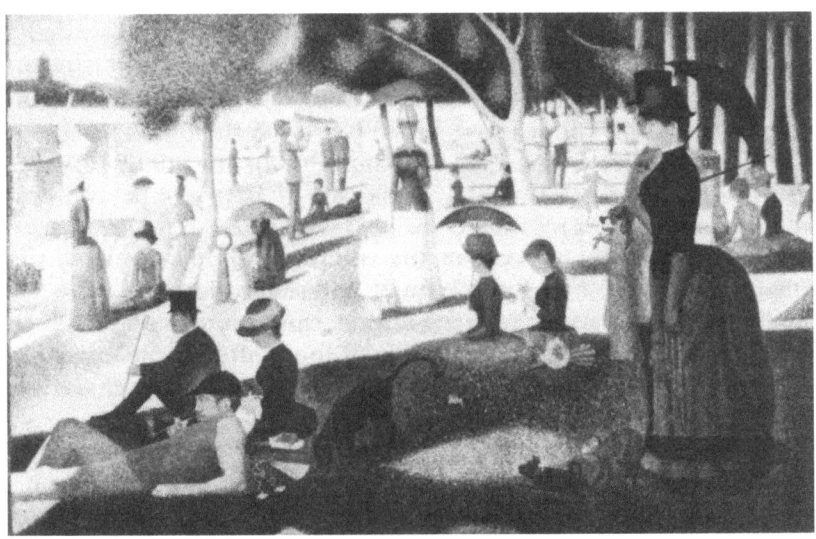

FIGURE 2.   Georges Seurat: "A Sunday Afternoon on the Island of La Grande Jatte" 1884–86. Oil on canvas, 6' 9½ " x 10' 1¼ ". The Art Institute of Chicago. Helen Birch Bartlett Memorial Collection.

ist's own self-transformational needs, I find it more than coincidental that Seurat was exploring "field" tensions artistically while James Maxwell, his British contemporary, was elaborating his field theory, which describes mathematically the distribution of particles in electric and magnetic fields. An intent viewer of Seurat's painting would actively assimilate a perception of the world, new to that time, that stressed the placement of particles in atomistic fields, their relation to one another, and the fields of force in which they interact. Seurat researched the world with concepts similar to those of Faraday and Maxwell, creating a kind of visual field theory on canvas; he also prepared us for their concepts and ordered thinking along novel perceptual lines. In the company of other artists of the modern period, he elicited perceptual activity that is analytic and reductionistic in its intention, that is, a perceptual stance similar to that of the activity of the research scientist.

It is hard to imagine that Seurat's work was seen by his contemporaries as outrageous and unacceptable. We recognize its greatness and puzzle over why anyone could take offense. In an age when the aesthetic assumptions of Impressionism and Post-Impressionism have been assimilated into our cultural selves, and to which perceptions we have accommodated our expectations, it is almost incredible to us to hear writers contemporary with the Impressionists denouncing their style. But, with our knowledge of the mechanics of resistance to innovation, we can understand typical criticism of the period, such as that of Max Nordau, who stated that the style resulted from the "nystagmus found in the eyes of 'degenerates' and the partial anesthesia of the retinal of hysterics" (quoted in Arnheim, 1971, p. 10).

From the perspective of our contemporary viewer, we shall note only a few of the multifaceted set of meanings expressed in this masterpiece, in which contradiction and the eloquent expression of opposing tendencies combine. In this work by a young artist (Seurat was 25 years old when he painted it), we see the boldness of invention and the intuitive genius with which he saw color and spatial relationships, which he used to create a style of expression still meaningful more than a century later.

We might, for example, point out the divergence between two coexisting spatial views of the work. In one of these, we attend to its flatness, planarity, and apparent two-dimensionality; this view is in marked contrast with another view, which takes in the expansive use of light and the pulsating porous quality of the membranous surface, which seems to breathe in color and sunshine, expanding spatial depth. The work's luminescence, however, is not that of Impressionism, whose reflections often conveyed the sense of the specific instant. Here we see Seurat's unique technique of showing color and light (in which he deliberately used the color principles of Helmholtz and Chevreul), which somehow conveyed a sense of suspension in time and movement. At first, the viewer takes in the particulars of the painting's language, the unique expression of color through the use of dots, the interplay between surface and depth, the nature of the picture space, and the tight, formal composition. Meaning is expanded as the painting's particulars are abstracted and universalized in a process inherent in perception (Arnheim, 1966).

Engagement with the perceptual ambiguities soon brings us to consider matters proximal to ourselves of a more personal, and, at the same time, of a more universal and abstract motif. For example, one could become involved in the dialectical play between the quality of that particular moment in time and the sense of the instantaneous eternal. Before long, we may find ourselves wondering about the instantaneous and the timeless in our own lives. The effect is one of silent stillness, a kind of photographic image in which the truth that inhabits each moment of existence has been caught for eternity. The painting portrays the universal and the timeless; yet the use of dots and the shimmering sunlit effect remind us, by contrast, of instant dissolution and fragmentation. The pointillist technique proclaims at once the constancy and yet the frailty of this seemingly serene and idyllic river-bank scene.

The illustration may be of a society threatened by atomistic dissolution; or, the ultimate effect produced in the viewer can be the opposite, the image of a society at rest. Using meticulously calculated color values, Seurat created a world in which each spatial element and each color has its place, so that the apparent spontaneity of a holiday afternoon is rigorously ordered and made part of a grand scheme. We are exquisitely in touch with the figures in the painting, of which the dots are component parts. We feel the tensions elaborated by the particular placement of each figure, like each dot, in a field where everything is related to its counterpart and nothing stands by itself. His technique, as well as his tight, formal composition, may entreat us to consider the broad sweep and order of our existence and its value in relationship to others. Through the highly ordered technique of the artist, we are able to apprehend order in our own lives in the midst of apparent disarray and random disorder.

What dialectical activity is recruited in us? It seems clear that in viewing the dots, we are called upon immediately to resolve the problem of their confluence and opposing discreteness. We are drawn into activity to mix the colors and separate them in our own way. We become acutely aware of the artist's technique, as we are involved in a technical activity ourselves. With each set of dots, and with our own efforts around them, we become more acutely attuned to the painter's work and allied with it, including his background theory, as we visually make color. We empathically join up with the self of the painter, with his artistic problems, and with his successes. That is, our consciousness joins up with the full symbolic expression of the work; as a consequence, we may feel an increasing empowerment to create order in our own lives, to seek the universal and timeless truths in each moment, and to synthesize the various forms of expression into the cohesive entity that Kohut calls the "cohesive-productive self." Most important, the painting expresses something about the transformation of the self, the self of the artist in evolving a mode of expression that goes beyond his Impressionist forebears, and the transformation of the self of the viewer in his experience of the work's rich visual meaning and the symbolic content he draws from the painting for his conceptual use.

Metapsychologically, what happens between us and the work? That is, what set of psychological functions does it have for us? A self at a lower condition of order, as it first encounters the work, will experience the frustration of an unfamiliar object whose language it is only partially attuned to. Prolonged immersion in the work produces frustration, which will decrease proportionately as the unraveling of the work's secrets render it more understandable. Increased understanding of the work may bring about in the viewer a sense of need satisfaction and increased cohesiveness, even exhilaration. The establishment of "empathic resonance" (Wolf, 1981) with a work's meaning will enhance the sense of cohesiveness, harmony, and positive affective coloring of the self. The mechanisms of accommodation and assimilation (Piaget and Inhelder, 1969) come into play. A viewer might, for example, assimilate features of the pointillist vision described earlier, ambiguously dividing colors carefully into their components and then re-fusing them into their shared hue. As he does this, he might accommodate his perceptions to look for similar ambiguities in other areas of color or composition, ultimately experimenting with accommodating his vision similarly in the world beyond the painting. With increasing comprehension, the work will become alive, and the world will also become enlarged with new possibilities. As a new way of organizing our visual stimuli becomes assimilated, our perceptions and our conceptions will both be transformed.

This type of interaction can take place with the formal aspects of a painting, as opposed to the narrative elements, and is further illustrated in abstract art, where narrative elements are absent. Take for example, the wholly abstract work "The Golden Wall" (Fig. 3), which was painted in the United States about 80 years after "La Grande Jatte." The artist was Hans Hofmann, the German-born art educator

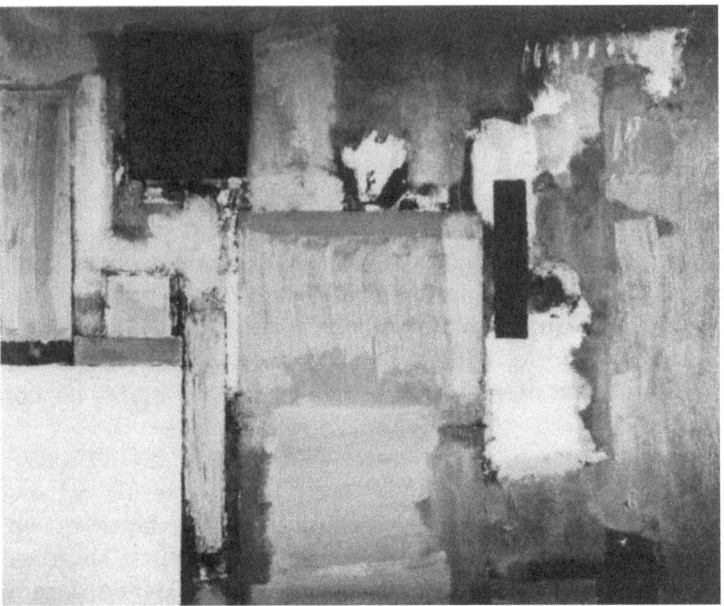

FIGURE 3.   Hans Hofmann: "The Golden Wall" 1961. 60" x 72". The
Art Institute of Chicago.

and Abstract Expressionist painter. In it are striking differences from
Seurat's work and also many thematic similarities, among them color
and light as important subjects of study. This painting is abstract because it does not illustrate a specific scene, and it is expressionist in
that the relationships of composition, color, and form are determined
by the inner need and feelings of the artist, and the painting projects
these. This great painting has it roots in the major painting traditions
of the century—Post-Impressionism, Fauvism, German Expressionism,
and French and American Cubism; but Hofmann has integrated and
transformed all of these into his own contribution. It is clearly Hofmann's statement, and it is instantly recognizable as such. We catch
its meaning, like that of any artwork, by giving ourselves over to interaction with it in dialogue with its elements, seen on their own terms.

In the "The Golden Wall," Hofmann is discussing, in the language
of painting, the properties of light and color. He is exploring many
of the polarities we reviewed with Seurat's work: the instant as opposed to the eternal, the ambiguity of picture surface and depth, and
the expressive potential of colors singly and in relation to one another.
As soon as we attempt to put these matters into words, however, we
realize how different are the languages spoken by these pictures, how
different are their modes of expression, and how different are vocabu-

laries with which they explore seemingly similar thematic terrain.

What do Hoffman's tough but subtle color expressions evoke in us? If we look at the dominant color, red, for a moment, we note that there is a gradation of reds of differing intensities, surfaces, color values, shapes, boundaries, and neighbors, all evoking contrasting and con- tradictory feelings in us. Red is an intense color, the color of flame, joyousness, expansiveness, and intensity of feeling, yet it also can have destructive and satanic connotations. The central declarative red rec- tangle has blue and yellow neighbors, which balance the intense ex- pansiveness of the central reds and set up pulsating, oscillating forces. Some colors, for example, take us forward, others backward, so that advance and recession forces are set up, while the colored masses sur- round newly created space. Hofmann's work expands on the explora- tion of the nature of the picture space and its definition by color. He explores how picture elements, such as planes of color, created expand- ing and contracting forces through their relation to one another. Univer- salized, his work can evoke the dynamic interrelationship of the elements of natural systems, a pictorial relativity theory as it were. His activity with color evokes in the viewer corresponding dynamic emo- tional tensions, and the painting soon invites us to feel with Hofmann a certain joy in the freedom to describe our inner feelings and ambiva- lences, albeit within the constraints of opposing forces and arbitrary perimeters. A feeling of *joie de vivre* is conveyed within the context of contrasting and ambiguous tensions.

In Seurat's work there is the interplay between static and dynamic forces. Similarly, the different elements in this abstract by Hofmann soon come to be seen in constant flux with each other, and each ele- ment is seen only insofar as it creates tension in another one. Seurat's exploration strikes us as more formal and cerebral. In Hofmann's paint- ing we do not look to the elements as through a proscenium onto a stage, but rather we are in immediate contact with the elements that appear almost to reach out and include us. Rather than the self–other dichotomy rendered more evident in the still stagelike formal arrange- ment of Seurat, Hofmann seems to include us, as we feel a certain play- ful invitation to participate in his painting. The surface values remind us of the physical separation between our physical self and the can- vas, but in one of those ambiguities central to the art experience, we oscillate between our awareness of the physical separation and the predominantly joyous merger the illuminating values of the canvas. Far more than the Seurat canvas, which made initial probes into this area, Hofmann's painting is highly personal. It celebrates the sentient self, the right of emotionality to be seen and heard on its own terms. These are certainly values with which any psychoanalyst can resonate.

Among other effects, the abstract mode of expression mightily increases the confidence of the viewer to possess his own expression of feelings and to evolve his own capacity to create order.

THEORETICAL DISCUSSION

Within Kohut's framework, how can the interaction with paintings be viewed? Psychologically speaking, the subjective sense of self is somehow coextensive with that of the work and therefore intrinsically with the artist's personality. The psychological boundaries of the self become merged with that of the painting, creating activity in the intervening and shared psychological space. The constituents of this space are the viewer's subjective psychological experience, his experience of the painting, the material reality of the painting itself, and the painter's artistic personality at that time. This is a live dynamic interactive psychological space. Communication goes on over time at multiple layers of fact, value, symbol, and feeling, at conscious and unconscious levels. My stress is on the less conscious aspects of perception (i.e., the formal qualities of art) that enable the conception of new organizing conceptual structures and also produce synthesis, unity, and coherence, rather than chaos and primitive disorder.[3]

One of the distinguishing features of the selfobject is that its boundaries do not end with the physical boundary of the self. The intrapsychic experience of the person is in a continuum with the elements oustide of itself; it surrounds and ingests, so to speak, the perceived responses of others out of need to use these responses in the service of the various selfobject needs of the self. This activity goes on continuously and is part of the automatic, hypothesizing activity of the self.

Embodied within this deceptively simple concept are processes of great complexity that occur in that area that includes the subject and object but is not restricted to either of them. The selfobject concept comprises what is out there, such as person, canvas, stage, screen, and yet it is coextensive with the individual psychological experience of the self. It denotes a self in the here and now but also faces forward in time and action, to a potential future uttering of its capabilities. At the height of aesthetic excitement, whether from the vantage point of viewer or of painter, the psychological barrier between self and other is nonexistent, and the painting, for example, is fused with one's experiencing self. We can imagine the fluidity between the self and the art object for the sake of artistic experience.

---

[3]It is interesting in this regard that the psychoanalytic literature on abstract art is relatively sparse, while that on narrative or figurative art is more abundant.

At first we might feel some opposition to this concept of fusion, since we are accustomed to picturing the self as having specific boundaries that are congruent with the physical boundaries of the person. Separation of self and object is customarily associated with maturation, whereas the merger of self and object has traditionally been associated with maturational failure, or regression to delusional infantile omnipotence (Milner, 1957; Finegarette, 1958). That self and object are often dynamically merged as an intergral part of mature, adult, everyday experience is an idea that may be greeted with resistance, especially as applied to cultural phenomena. Self–object merger is described in the psychoanalytic literature mainly perjoratively, with implications for pathological symbiosis and psychotic regression (see, for example, the "unio mystica" concept of Fenichel, 1945).

The area where self encounters object is important, since so much of the literature about creativity, from both within and outside of psychoanalysis, has placed the creative process and its apprehension at that boundary area where self and object are fused, merged, or otherwise in contact with one another. Winnicott's (1971) seminal idea of the "transitional object" refers to this illusionary merger, and it is in the area of the "potential space" (p. 126) between baby and mother that Winnicott located creative play and cultural experience. This space is formed in the area that exists between baby and mother as separation of self and object occur in the process of maturation. Nevertheless, in Winnicott's theory, this potential space remained transitional from one developmental phase to another, and the object relations theory associated with him does not go on to explain fully how creative experience, including cultural and ritualistic events, can occur in a space that one is optimally expected to grow out of. Milner (1957) focuses on the same area in her seminal book on art. Bollas (1978), influenced by Winnicott, feels that aesthetic experiences induce an "existential recollection" of the time when the mother provided the infant with an experience of continuity and being. Rose (1980) comes close to the selfobject concept when he discusses how art catalyzes the techniques by which the ego shapes and simplifies its world. The selfobject concept advances our understanding that fusions of self and other experiences exist as part of the psychology of everyday life, without requiring us to reroute them, as it were, through waystations of pathology, psychosis, or infantile narcissism. The concept of the selfobject in psychoanalysis allows us to integrate artistic experience systematically into metapsychology. Fusion of self and object is not necessarily archaic, primitive, regressive, hallucinatory, or paranoid, but it can be any of these and necessitates a discussion of optimal psychical distance.

In art, distance gives perspective and facilitates critical judgment. Psychodynamically, it represents the other pole in that alternating interplay of fusion and separation with the art object. This movement between different positions of observation is the "antinomy of distance" (Bullough, 1912). In art it represents the different vantage points from which we might view any work. We psychologically shift back and forth between poles of underdistance and overdistance, positioning ourselves in ambiguous and changing relationship to the content of the work. Our vantage point is mobile and fluid rather than fixed.

From the artist's point of view, if a work is overdistanced, it may be overintellectualized and therefore sterile; if it is underdistanced, such as in the autistic drawings of schizophrenic artists, too much of the personal torment of the artist, no matter how skilled he is, may be portrayed to allow aesthetic abstraction. Looking at it from a selfobject point of view, we might say that optimal distance is dependent on the fit between the two conjoined subjectivities of viewer and art work, of self and selfobject. Underdistancing, with the breakthrough of drive products into behavior (e.g., the viewer slashes the canvas) would be formulated as a rupture in the intersubjective integrity of the selfobject relationship, with the emergence of distorted or pathologically exaggerated instinctual behavior as "breakdown products" of a fragmented selfobject relationship. Optimal distance is that in which useful perception and its universalizing consequence, symbolic activity, occurs.

Discussing psychological space highlights that psychological activity in which symbols are created. Symbolic activity arises out of the need of the individual to create useful relationships between inner and outer conditions for the sake of adaptation to these conditions. Such activity occurs in a psychological space that allows the blending of known and foreign elements, so that order, knowledge, and mastery can occur. We can, for example, place elements "out there" in the world, to try to make it known; for example, a penis may be seen as swordlike or crosslike. Similarly, we can use known elements in the self to make outside experience intelligible; for example, a sword or a cross may be seen as penislike. This activity, in which the art object acts as selfobject, is the process by which symbol formation occurs. The selfobject, through its emphasis on shared, communicative space, makes the process of creating symbols more understandable.

An outcome of the special focus on the spatial qualities of the selfobject was the formulation of the concept of the "intersubjective field" (Brandchaft and Stolorow, 1983), that is, the psychological field in which two participating subjective psychological realities intersect. The intersubjective space designates that psychological arena in which the aesthetic show goes on. Thomson (1984) has described the intersubjective area as a field of communication in which there are qualities of "interlocking responsivity" and sensitive attunments in cognitive and affective exchanges. Closely tuned intersubjective communication also occurs in art. Insofar as a painting "talks" to us, we hear its voice, listen to its language in the shared space occupied by the viewer's unique receptivity and the symbolic expressions offered in condensed form in the painting. As in dialogue, the activity of the viewer acquaints him, through active attention, empathy, and searching contemplation, with the condensed, contrasting, and often ambiguous aesthetic meanings consolidated into the forms portrayed.[4]

The study of the symbolic function particularly highlights the ability of art objects, redolent with symbols bearing affective and cognitive significance, to serve as selfobjects for the self. In general, the pursuit of artistic involvement is carried out by a self possessing some level of need, minor or urgent, for enhanced self-organization; the hoped for response is through the dialectic with the art work, whether as viewer or creator. This acquisition of personal order is what Arnheim alluded to in his work. As Milner (1957) says, "Are we not rather driven by the internal necessity for inner organization, pattern, coherence, the basic need to discover identity and difference, without which the experience becomes chaos?" (p. 182). The selfobject concept is a suitable one for embedding the process of metaphoric experience. A painting, however free of naturalistic representation, always has psychological symbolic content, and it can be said to be functioning as a work of art insofar as it functions symbolically.

So far, we have discussed the space in which selfobject functioning occurs and the oscillation between "merger" and "distance" that characterizes it. Now let us examine the way in which art objects can provide ordering information that enhances the process of symbol formation. Selfobject functioning includes the known classical categories of mirroring, idealizing, and twinship. The process I shall describe, which I designate as "transformational functioning," is not separate from these but instead provides the microstructure for them all. Rather mirroring's enhancement of self-cohesion, transformational activity denotes the specific details of the ordering (cognitive) information transmitted during mirroring processes. In the next section I shall explore this idea, illustrating it in art and discussing some developmental aspects of it.

The relationship in question is between a self at a lesser order of organization and a selfobject that aids in its higher order structuralization by providing information or symbolic interchange, that is, through the reception into the organization of the self of specific information. The process alters the self-experience and enables metamorphosis to higher levels of organization and development. "Informa-

---

[4]Gombrich (1954) has described the importance of the role of ambiguity in setting up the dialectic to which aesthetic emotion is the heir.

tion," taken literally, means giving form, and it is defined here as any sensory datum that induces order. The self's immediate experience is based in the relationship with a selfobject that functions by providing ordering information aligned with the order-seeking needs of the self. The data received provide ordering information about our basic categories of organizing experience, that is, about space, time, number, and causality. These are the data the active mind uses to construct its reality. What distinguishes this mode of selfobject functioning is that information—a word, a glance, a spatial concept, an instruction, an imparted level of energy, a particular tone, beat, or rhythm, a certain level of expressed vitality (Stern, 1985)—all order experience and allow the recipient the chance of a higher order adaptation to its milieu. This "transformational" activity is transmitted to the self through the functional responses of the selfobject. The classical modes of selfobject functioning (mirroring, idealization, and the like) are intertwined with and depend on transformational activity; indeed, they seem to represent the larger functional categories for which transformational activity provides the basic grammar and through which it is uttered. This interpretive functioning of the selfobject answers the needs of the self throughout life, as the person seeks a way of ordering his often mystifying world for the purpose of growth and change. As Ornstein (1980) has pointed out (in writing about the concept of psychological health), there is a continual process of the unfolding of the self's intrinsic patterns in the pursuit of a "higher order concept of adaptation", that is, the realization of the self's embryonic potential for higher development.

The artistic enterprise conducts, facilitates, and catalyses transformational processes at multiple levels of complexity. Close inspection of the artistic process reveals the importance of transformational activity and its effects as a fashioner of guiding values. The artist, through his carefully conceived and crafted works, and employing his own style, conveys a complex network of feelings and concepts that recruits complementary feelings in us and shapes our attitude toward the work and ultimately toward the world. For parallel work within the domain of cognitive psychology, see Gombrich (1984), Bruner (1984), Arnheim (1966). They underline the impossibility of separating perception on the one hand from hypothesizing and problem-solving on the other. These findings join up with those of psychoanalytic research in which tachistoscopic techniques were used to explore the unconscious effects of subliminally delivered stimuli (Silverman, 1978, for example.) While paintings as such are not subliminal stimuli, their perceptual and symbolic contents operate largely out of the range of awareness until interpretation perhaps makes them conscious.

Thus, art brings the viewer's effortful activity into the picture (though the activity may be largely nonconscious). Each viewer becomes a cocreator (Kris, 1952). To the extent that the viewer then discovers, with the artist, unified, coherent, solutions to the problems presented, he experiences an acquisition of useful information. The word "information" does not-do justice to the complexity and three-dimensionality of the data received, which is often purveyed simultaneously through multiple channels, for example, color as well as scale and texture. The data may be at once perceptual, cognitive, affective, instinctual, and spiritual. The word "wisdom" conveys better the subjective experience accompanying the accretion of complex symbolic meanings. Man's cognitive capacities enable him to conceive the universal and the particular at the same moment and to oscillate back and forth between these two levels of significance. Art stimulates the mind into hypothesizing and patterning activity, and the viewer, who is brought into that activity, can then feel enlightened as his capacity to find order is universalized by his immersion in the symbolic action of the work. Oremland (1984) refers to this as the "parsimonious dialectic with universals" that gives art its enduring power.

In this discussion, we have attended mostly to the viewer of art, but similar processes can also be described in the area of interaction between the artist and his own work. He puts his own puzzles and internal ambiguities outside of himself and then reacts to them as if they were other than his. In a sense, once the artist begins a work, he surrenders to it as though the work were dominating him, demanding the solution of its own ambiguities, and requiring completion. The artist experiences the selfobject functioning of the art work as alive, active, interpretive, and eventually having transformational capabilities, to the extent that the inner puzzles of the artist are worked out through this externalization. Ehrenzweig (1967), working from a Kleinian framework, has looked at this externalization process in detail. Using different terminology, the process he describes parallels in many ways to the process of transmuting internalization described by Kohut, (1983) except that Ehrenzweig's concepts fail to remove the creative process from the psychopathologizing concepts with which it remains pejoratively enmeshed.

Transformational functions characterize the creative process in artists and in the audience they address. Resistances to transformational activity are intrinsic to that process, just as resistances to the interpretive process occur in psychoanalytic treatment. In the artistic arena, what are the resistances, if any, against being the object of transformational resistances? The community expression of such resistance can be seen in the protest and outrage that often attend the first exhibition of original work. Art work utilizing underlying assumptions beyond the prevailing, culturally affirmed ones may be rejected as unacceptable on varying grounds. One historical example is the ecclesiastical efforts to dress Michelangelo's nudes in the Sistine Chapel ceiling. We can be amused now that Jackson Pollock was known as "Jack the Dripper" when his famous pour and drip masterpieces first appeared. Defensive denial, disavowal, or distortion of the perceptual input are the consequences of transformational resistances. In the art field, this can result in the discarding of works seen to be great only by later generations, when the significant truths of the art works can be more comfortably received. The cool, infused light of Vermeer's interiors had to wait two centuries for recognition of their greatness. It seems that, at first, underlying assumptions of new art are absorbed and psychologically worked over at unconscious levels over time. The "I get it!" phenomenon may lag far behind a viewer's initial contact with a work, sustained until comprehension occurs. The artist's researches into alternative ways of viewing space, time, causality, and the like provide the background to what Kohut (1977) called the "hypothesis of artistic anticipation" (pp. 285–286), that is, that the great artist is ahead of his time in focusing on the nuclear psychological problems of his era.

Thus, transformational activity denotes the microstructure of communication, in which specific cognitive information is conveyed with subsequent ordering effects on the self's interpretations of the world. Transformational activity is intertwined with the experience of selfobjects and relies on the experience of responsiveness and attunement inherent in this process. The effect of such cognitive information is to enable the self to arrive at a higher level of self-organization through the accretion of increased information about space, time, form, and causality. This process is particularly evident in the processes occurring in art and is given recognition by the cultural and political prominence art occupies.

One objection to using the selfobject concept in this instance is that a selfobject cannot be an inanimate object. This objection is refuted by the recognition that in the distinctively aesthetic experience, the self is influenced through its dialectic with the condensed symbolic assertions of the art object and therefore with those of the person of the artist who created it. In other words, the selfobject functioning of the art work, at the moments that constitute the aesthetic experience, is constituted not by the material qualities of the object, but by the condensed communication of tensions provoked by the symbolic—therefore human—assertions of the work. It is not the art work's material objecthood that induces the aesthetic experiences and the formative influences that derive from them; the pigment and canvas themselves do not organize the self. Rather, the symbolized contents invite the viewer's response, be it only repudiation. The interplay is quite human, even though the particular medium that fosters it is inanimate. In fact, the material objecthood of the work, its material qualities, is contradictory to its aesthetic potential.

The question has been asked whether extending the selfobject concept to inanimate objects trivializes the concept, renders it insignificant. Trivialization could occur only if the concept failed to distinguish between ideas where a signifier of importance is needed. If the concept of the selfobject is applied to a very wide range of experiences, for example, the fender of one's car to a beach chair, it can lose its power as a concept to distinguish between more or less significant events for the self. If, while driving in a fog, one feels subjectively more secure by the clear perception of the position of one's left fender, does this relatively simple signal function serve as a selfobject function? Surely one must distinguish between a signal experience and the aesthetic experience on the basis of depth and complexity. I have already pointed out that the selfobject is not actual pigment and canvas but the contained symbolic meanings that are pertinent. To insist that the application of the selfobject concept to art trivializes it fails to take into account the rich, multi-dimensional and multi-layered quality of the aesthetic experience and the full measure of its cognitive and affective complexities. The complex, symbolic contents of the art work, even more than in a dream, lend themselves to interpretation (and therefore to dialogue) from many points of view—historical, iconographic, cultural, formal, technical, libidinal. This rich complexity of indwelling symbolism permits exchange that is more in keeping with what we have come to regard as selfobject functioning. A signal may alter one's percepts for a moment; an art work can sculpt one's values for a lifetime.

Rather than the selfobject concept of artistic functioning being a trivialization, it is a challenge to extend the clinical concept of the selfobject to enrich our understanding of the complexities of human psychology beyond the clinical sphere. By seeing psychoanalysis as the science of complex human states, we can apprehend in aesthetic functioning complex states beyond what might be describable in the clinical situation, since the materials unique to the artistic situation do not ordinarily present themselves in the consulting room, or, if they do, they require a kind of analysis that might not occur. Limitations presented by the preeminence of clinical goals or the aesthetic limitations of the analyst or patient may prevent the full unfolding of the selfobject potential of human experience. There might be a dimension of psychological experience accessible only in the gallery or studio. Could it be that the artistic experience thus reminds us of the (narcissistically, to the analyst) injurious idea that the clinical arena "trivializes" to some extent the full breadth and dimensionality of human potential experience, and that the fullest aspects of cognitive, affective, and spiritual experience also lie beyond the reach of clinical psychoanalytic grasp?

REFERENCES

Arnheim, R. (1966), *Toward a Psychology of Art.* Los Angeles: University of California Press.
Arnheim, R. (1971) *Entropy and Art.* Berkeley: University of California Press.
Barr, A., Jr., (1946), *Picasso: Fifty Years of His Art.* New York: Museum of Modern Art.
Basch, M. (1975), Toward a theory that encompasses depression: A revision of existing causal hypotheses in psychoanalysis. In: *Depression and Human Existence,* ed. E. J. Anthony & T. Benedek. Boston: Little, Brown, pp. 485–534.
Berenson, B. (1950), *Aesthetics and History.* London, England: Constable.
Brandchaft, B. & Stolorow, R. (1983), Development and pathogenesis: An intersubjective viewpoint. Unpublished paper.
Bollas, C. (1978), The aesthetic moment and the search for transformation. *The Annual of Psychoanalyis,* 6:385–394. New York: International Universities Press.
Bruner, J. (1984), Interaction, communication and self. *J. Amer. Acad. Child Psychiat.,* 23:1–7
Bullough, E. (1912), "Psychical distance" as a factor in art and an aesthetic principle. *Brit. J. Psychol.,* 5:87–98.
Ehrenzweig, A. (1967), *The Hidden Order of Art.* Berkeley: University of California Press.
Fenichel, O. (1945), *The Psychoanalytic Theory of Neurosis.* New York: Norton.
Finegarette, H. (1958), The ego and mystic selflessness. *Psychoanal. Rev.,* 45:5–41.
Freud, S. (1914), The Moses of Michelangelo. *Standard Edition,* 13:211–236. London: Hogarth Press, 1953.
Gedo, J. (1979), *Beyond Interpretation.* New York: International Universities Press.
Gombrich, E. (1954), Psychoanalysis and the history of art. *Internat. J. Psycho-Anal.,* 35:401–411.
Kandinsky, W. (1912), *Concerning the Spiritual in Art.,* trans. M. Sadler. New York: Dover, 1977.
Kohut, H. (1976), Creativeness, charisma, and group psychology: Reflections on the self-analysis of Freud. In: *The Search for the Self, Vol. 2,* ed. P. Ornstein. New York: International Universities Press, 1978, pp. 793–843.
———— (1977), *The Restoration of the Self.* New York: International Universities Press.
———— (1983), *How Does Analysis Cure?* ed. A. Goldberg. Chicago: University of Chicago Press.
Kris, E. (1952), *Psychoanalytic Explorations in Art.* New York: International Universities Press.
Milner, M. (1957), *On Not Being Able to Paint.* New York: International Universities Press.
Oremland, J. (1984), Empathy and its relation to the appreciation of art. In: *Empathy I,* ed. J. Lichtenberg, M. Bornstein & D. Silver. Hillsdale, NJ: The Analytic Press, pp. 239–266.
Ornstein, P. (1980), Self psychology and the concept of health. In: *Advances in Self Psychology,* ed. A. Goldberg. New York: International Universities Press.
Piaget, J. & Inhelder, B. (1969), *The Psychology of the Child.* New York: Basic Books.
Rose, G. (1980), The power of form. *Psychological Issues,* Monogr. 49. New York: International Universities Press.

Rotenberg, C. (1985), A psychoanalytic study of the appreciation of art. *J. Amer. Acad. Psychoanal,* 13:113–127.

——— (1984), Selfobject theory and the artistic process. Presented at meeting of Toronto Psychoanalytic Society.

Silverman, S. (1978), The "innate givens": A reconsideration in relation to some specific psychotic phenomena. Unpublished study.

Stern, D. N. (1985), *The Interpersonal World of the Infant.* New York: Basic Books.

Thomson, P. G. (1984), Analysis as an intersubjective field of communication. Presented at meeting of Toronto Psychoanalytic Society, Nov.

Weissman, P. (1971), The artist and his objects. *Internat. J. Psycho-Anal.* 52:401–406.

Winnicott, D. (1971), The place where we live. In: *Playing and Reality.* New York: Penguin.

Wolf, E. (1981), Empathic resonance. Presented at the Fourth Conference on Self Psychology. Berkeley, CA.

Chapter 14

Treatment of Narcissistic Vulnerability in Marital Therapy

Marion F. Solomon

Where marriages are made up of individuals with self disorders, it is crucial that therapeutic treatments be developed that take into account the fragile, easily damaged self of one or both partners. An important goal of therapy is to help each partner hear and respond to the needs of the injured self of the other.

SELF AND OTHER
IN INTIMATE RELATIONSHIPS

Two variables influence the course of all intimate relationships; 1) differentiation and autonomy, and 2) the wish for a symbiotic, mergerlike state of at-one-ment in which there is perfect understanding by a loving other. Finding a balance between these two wishes that is acceptable to both partners is the quandary facing love relationships (Solomon, 1988).

Many family therapists contend that treatment should be designed to help the family move as rapidly as possible toward increased differentiation, and that each new gain in individuality brings the togetherness forces to a higher level of adaptation (Bowen, 1972, 1976). But to presume a hierarchy of health and pathology based on the concept of differentiation leaves out the normal need for selfobjects throughout life. Kohut (1977) notes that although they normally evolve from archaic into more mature forms, some need for selfobjects remain in everyone. He writes "there is no mature love in which the love object is not also a selfobject . . . to put this depth-psychological formulation into a psychosocial context: There is no love relationship without mutual, self-esteem enhancing, mirroring and idealization" (p. 122).

PATTERNS OF NARCISSISTIC VULNERABILITY IN MARRIAGE

Healthy marriages succeed partly because the partners are able to gratify their spouse's needs for idealizing and mirroring. These needs are mature to the extent that they are both realistic and limited. Each partner realizes that the spouse is a separate individual with important needs of his or her own. Both also know that functioning as a selfobject for their mates does not mean that their own needs will be interfered with, diminished, scorned, or overlooked. They recognize unconsciously that childhood needs for idealization and mirroring are never fully outgrown. Both partners are able to tolerate in themselves and in their mates temporary and limited regressions. Healthy marriages thus include the freedom to regress to "mutual childlike dependency in flexible role exchanges" (Dicks, 1967).

As I read Kohut's description of selfobject needs of mirroring, idealizing, and twinship, I could not help but think of the couples whom I see in conjoint marital therapy. While their presenting problems center around specific issues such as money, work, sex or children, at a deeper level, couples are often dealing with narcissistic vulnerability and selfobject failures of partners for each other.

A good marriage flourishes partly because the partners gratify each other's infantile needs. The desire for another who functions as an unconditional mirror and the tendency to adore another as an ideal are mature insofar as they are coupled with realistic expectations of reciprocity and as long as they are limited in duration. If marriage partners recognize, consciously or unconsciously, that some childhood needs are never completely outgrown, each spouse can function as a "selfobject" for the other without feeling diminished.

Everyone needs somebody else's support from time to time. A person suffering from early injuries, however, lacks the empathy necessary to see another as a separate individual with his or her own needs. Indeed, confirmation of the grandiose fantasy of fusion requires control of the partner. The need for control is often accompanied by the fear of the partner's anger and by fear of abandonment. People whose vulnerabilities arise from the failure of early relationships to accommodate primary narcissistic feelings end up depending excessively on others to provide coherence in their lives.

These patterns usually include a propensity to regress when there is a perceived threat to psychic functioning and a tendency toward domination by urgent archaic selfobject needs. When this occurs, others are experienced only as part of the self and are used to service and repair the disabled self. While such an experience may happen even to satisfactorily functioning persons in situations of great stress or embarrassment, certain people are prone to fragmentation and regressions.

Narcissistically vulnerable persons clearly are not prime candidates for intimate relationships (including therapy). They believe that they are always giving to others and are constantly disappointed that others do not reciprocate. They fail to recognize that what they do for others is based on their own desires, not on what others want. They have great difficulty listening to their partners and responding empathically. Instead, they are busy communicating their own wishes and finding ways to make their partners accommodate them. The result is that the partner feels oppressed and enslaved by the other's narcissistic expectations and demands.

Clearly there is a wide range of narcissistic vulnerability, from the occasional shame and embarrassment that anyone may feel in an extremely uncomfortable situation, to the proneness to injury and disorganization that occurs when there is a break in immediate need fulfillment. Therapists who work with marital problems encounter mates who fall anywhere along the continuum of health to pathology. Some people who are quite clearly disturbed nevertheless have successful marriages, whereas other people, who display no evidence of severe emotional problems, are involved in disastrous marriages (Solomon, 1985).

WHAT HAPPENS WHEN THE HONEYMOON IS OVER?

Romantic love in many ways resembles the very earliest relationships and archaic selfobject needs. In adulthood, lovers find in the reflection of the other's gaze a sense of being enjoyed, appreciated, affirmed, special, unique, and loved. Lang (1985) notes that ''there is a driving passion in new love which overcomes reason, logic, and the wish to be a separate autonomous person.''

To the extent that there were abuses, traumas, or chronic disappointment experienced in early life, the "child" in the adult relationship
of intimacy will tend to replay some kernel of early relationship—but
this time with the hope of repair. There is a wish to find "someone"
with whom to identify and a hope of acquiring the kind of power and
strength that the other represents.

A tendency to repeat early object relationships operates in all of us.
Those people who are fortunate enough to make good choices in their
lovers may find that the intimate relationship heals deficiencies in meeting some basic needs. Those whose choices are not so well fitting or
whose early failures are greater than the capacity of their partners to
overcome, may find themselves endlessly recreating the attempt at
wholeness through a reparative fusion with a partner. Lang (1985)
postulates that there is a "false recognition signal," a key piece found
in the lover, who in most ways may be very different than what is
wished for consciously. This key piece is the legacy of an early internalized object that serves as a reminder and results in an almost chem-
ical reaction that draws the lovers together.

In a loving relationship it is possible for the partners to develop a
mutual interplay and reciprocity with each other that, while imperfect
and subject to the usual stress of living together, may still provide for
both a way to be good selfobjects for one another, legitimizing their
own archaic needs by developing methods of caring for each other.
The result is that they become more tolerant of existing archaic needs,
both in their partner and in themselves (Solomon, 1988).

For most people, and certainly for those who seek therapy to help
their relationship, the partners have not been able to adequately provide this selfobject function for each other. The result is a great deal
of unhappiness and generally a symptom in at least one of the partners or their children.

BASIC SELF AND FUNCTIONING SELF

Therapists need to make diagnoses of health or pathology on the basis of the overall functioning of the individual. A functioning self,
however, is much more than health or pathology; it is a combination
of endowment, early interactions, and current relations with important others. A functioning self may be affected by stresses, anxiety,
and subjective reactions to others. When early life experiences have
resulted in a cohesive sense of self, a person is less likely to need to
borrow emotional strength from others.

If the individual sense of self is less than optimal, each partner in
a relationship may still find strength in the other and the functioning

self might operate at a very high level. In addition, having a good self-object relationship may, over time, provide a reparative experience that raises the level of the basic self. In such a relationship, two persons, each with narcissistic vulnerabilities that are pathological, may still complement each other. This may result in a reduction of chronic anxiety and change the way each of the partners interacts with the other and with members of the family. The result may be that the intensity of clinical symptoms decreases.

I believe that there is a way to work with couples that is reparative for narcissistically vulnerable persons. I am speaking of a psycho-dynamic therapeutic stance in which there is a strong focus on an empathic understanding of the interactional behavior of the partners and an awareness of transference reactions as they emerge between the partners and between each one and the therapist. It requires that the therapeutic setting be a safe, containing environment in which previously unacceptable feelings are allowed to be put on the table and discussed.

TREATMENT GOALS

The goals of marital therapy with couples who have self disorders vary depending upon the degree of narcissistic vulnerability of each partner and the history of injury in interaction between the pair. If a relationship has had a pattern of repeated injuries, there is little reservoir of good will and a limited willingness to trust each other with areas of vulnerability. The therapist must take an active stance as container and holder of communication between the partners. There is little advantage in encouraging partners to talk directly to each other when their messages are meant to attack and defend against each other. A new communicative language may have to be learned.

A longer term goal may be to increase tolerance of selfobject failures so that they no longer cause fears of loss of cohesion. The structures of the self may be developed to the point where there is a gradual replacement of the need for selfobjects with a firmed-up self and its functions. While this goal is more likely to require individual psychotherapy, I have worked with couples who, through a willingness to allow partners to share heretofore cut-off aspects of themselves, have learned to provide for each other an ongoing, safe, nontraumatic environment with only occasional failures. This provides opportunities for what Kohut (1971) calls "transmuting internalizations" to take place within the structure of the self. Transmuting internalizations are the internal changes that occur as the individual increasingly becomes able to accept the hurts that are caused by failures of optimal responses by important others.

Where the narcissistic vulnerability is not so great, couples can be taught how to become better selfobjects for each other through mirroring and idealizing responses to each other by learning to tolerate the less traumatic small failures of responses.

TREATMENTS

If the goal is a healing of the central disturbance and development of a cohesive self, it is very important for the therapist to avoid instructions that suggest changes in actions or behavior toward each other. This may at first seem impossible when one or both partners make overly demanding claims or expectations. The common sense response of the therapist may well be that such demands should be relinquished and reality limitations be made clear. Unfortunately, such a response may be perceived as a negative intrusion and experienced as a narcissistic injury.

It is important for the therapist to recognize that overly demanding expectations are part of the symptoms of narcissistic pathology. The essence of these patients is that access to the early narcissism is barred, and development of the self may depend on their getting in touch with, expressing, and learning to accept aspects of themselves that are buried and "guarded by a wall of shame and vulnerability" (Kohut and Wolf, 1978, p. 423). Censuring behavior, making in depth psychological interpretations, or making suggestions for new behavior that raise levels of anxiety may cause a defensive closing up, a burial or repression of narcissistic assertiveness, and an increase in the split in the personality. Often, a defensive mobilization of the archaic grandiose self may occur (the best defense is a good offense), thus escalating the destructive, attacking interactions of the couple.

Whether imposed by the mate or the therapist, a series of narcissistic injuries will make treatment lose its value. This is why the use of paradox—although valuable in work with neurotics who have a more solid sense of self—is contraindicated with narcissistically vulnerable patients. The defense against perceived attacks may increasingly become a resistance to treatment.

DEVELOPMENT OF
NARCISSISTIC TRANSFERENCE

Therapists who have observed my work with couples often comment on the extremely slow pace of the sessions, the repetitive patterns of interaction between the individuals, the couple, and the therapist. Expectations, demands, and questions are repeated by the couple, and persistent pressure placed on partner and on the therapist to react in a certain expected manner, the same "buttons pushed," hurts inflicted, hurried withdrawal, or scathing rage emerging.

Often there is the repeated turning to the partner or to the therapist for approval or confirmation that they are lovable, wonderful, special in some way. When confirmation is not immediately forthcoming, a deflation, and lethargic disappointment can be seen.

The role of the therapist is to focus not on the content but on the process of messages transmitted during the session. Therapeutic interventions in the communicative process may include examining with the mates the minute details of feelings as they emerge at points where anger arises; asking about what each expects when there are withdrawal, attack, and defense patterns; asking how they mobilize to protect themselves when they are feeling vulnerable. Depending upon the issues for the couple, these explorations may help to clarify the needs of each partner and allow them to recognize areas that are being protected.

Demands for praise and approval from one partner or both must be reexamined in this light. It is not a question of what is to be reasonably expected, but rather of what underlying needs one is wishing the partner to meet. Is it the desperate need of the unresponded-to child that is coming out in the relationship? Can the therapist comment on the patient's vulnerability with an empathic understanding of how frightening and hurtful it is to face that need? Can the partner be taught and given modeling for understanding that what might appear on the surface to be an attack or demand is actually the exposure of an area of exquisite sensitivity, helplessness, or hopelessness of ever having needs met? The therapist can help couples reinterpret anger, to recognize that rage may stem from an inability to assert needs and demands effectively.

When needs are allowed to be accepted freely, without judgment, and are understood empathically by the therapist, and then by the partner, the time may come when the narcissistically vulnerable persons become more accepting of themselves. It is the ability of the partners to overcome their need to hide shameful embarrassing feelings from each other that allows them to relinquish repression of archaic narcissistic needs. The therapist assists in this process by constantly reinterpreting content interactions to reflect underlying needs, for example, "Of course you are angry—you got hurt by what was said." The goal is not to change behavior, but to reunite disavowed parts of the self and to aid in the reemergence of narcissistic aspects: "You know that you are not siamese twins joined at the head, but you cannot help wishing that she could read your mind and understand you perfectly."

Couples can hear and understand these needs as they emerge, an understanding made easier by the tendency of people to choose mates at the same psychological level. The underlying needs may be very similar even if the way they are presented differ. She may smother while he withdraws—yet both are terrified of intimacy. She may infantilize in her nurturing; he may demand constant filling; both are ravenously hungry emotionally.

Patients are relieved to learn what their mate's behavior and statements really mean once they understand that the behavior is not meant as an attack but as a way of protecting against hurt. With this awareness, couples may be able to change patterns of defense and retaliation. As understanding increases and defenses are reduced, partners may come to be remarkably responsive to each other over time.

The therapy sessions at first are a haven where the partners are able to interact, knowing that here their discussions will not turn into destructive attacks. As they are able to hear each other at a deeper level, they begin to go home from sessions better able to serve selfobject functions for each other. Feeling or receiving empathic responses to previously submerged frightening feelings makes responsiveness to the partner easier. When it becomes less necessary to mobilize defenses against old needs and feelings, there may be a transformation of the self. Narcissistic demandingness may be replaced by normal assertiveness. Timidity and withdrawal from the partner used to protect against grandiose fantasies that would cause shame and embarrassment may be replaced by a willingness to expose high aspirations and devotion to ideals, as well as a joyful acceptance of healthy childhood grandiosity.

CASE ILLUSTRATION

Donna and Ivan are in their late forties and have been married for 18 years. Both products of entertainment business families, they often congratulated themselves on their successful relationship amid friends for whom broken marriages and serial monogamy are the norm.

Ivan was particularly pleased that Donna had never wanted to do the "women's lib thing" and contented herself with caring for him and their three children and shopping or entertainment.

About a year ago their marriage seemed to be falling apart. Donna began making demands—she wanted to start a business. She asked Ivan to leave and said she was going to get a divorce. Three times he left and then talked her into a reconciliation.

The third time she decided she needed either a divorce attorney or a marital therapist. She called for a consultation, saying that she doubted that Ivan would come in. I suggested that she tell her husband that the best way to work on improving their marriage was for both of them to come in together for a session. I made an appointment with her and said that I would see them together if they both were willing to come together. On the appointed day, Ivan came 15 minutes early and waited for Donna.

PROCESS NOTES	DISCUSSION
T: Can you tell me something about why you came to see me today and what you hope will happen here?	I ask questions that are open ended enough to allow them to give information about the problem and to demonstrate the way that they interact together. I listen for precipitating factors, long-term interaction, and historical factors about early relationships that affect current problems.
[Ivan begins by talking about how successful their marriage has been and how until a year ago Donna and he had only the usual kinds of problems.]	
I: We've had our problems but we've really been pretty content.	
D: You've been content. I'm not. I don't like the way you treat me.	As they respond, I watch their process as well as content: who begins, how do they respond, do they listen to each other, how they react when they disagree or feel hurt by what is said by the other. Eye contact with each is very important early in the therapy. I address my comment to both at the same time by speaking to Ivan and including Donna in my remarks, then turning to Donna to complete the thought.
I: I don't treat you any different than I always have.	
T: Perhaps we should take a look at what Donna means and what she doesn't like, and what you mean, Ivan, when you say you treat her as you always have.	
D: I'm tired of taking care of you all the time. I'm tired of not having a life of my own.	
I: You've got a terrific life. I do all the work and you just go to lunch and shop.	
T: Perhaps that is part of the problem. Donna says she feels that she has no life of her own. She is angry that you don't hear her. You don't know what that means— things seem okay to you, yet she complains.	I do not respond to the problem presented until I can say something about the issues of both. I then speak of what I understand each has been describing: the confusion and frustration that Ivan feels, and the angry demands for a self of her own from Donna. Donna gives a piece of the unwritten marriage contract. He supports the family and has a right to let his anger out freely. She supports him emotionally and accepts his moods without
I: Well, what does she want? She can do anything she wants.	
D: I don't want to be married to you. I don't need to put up with what you do. You do everything you feel like and everyone jumps	

and if we don't you scream at us. Well, I'm not doing that anymore. I hate your temper tantrums.

I: I just blow off steam sometimes. I don't mean anything by it. I never hurt anyone.

D: You keep losing secretaries. They don't like it either. You have no right to scream at me like you do.

I: You're my wife, not some dumb secretary. We have a good marriage. What about our kids? It's not good for me to leave.

D: The kids are afraid of you. They don't ever want to talk to you.

I: They are teenagers. They have their own life. They don't talk much to you either.

T: Okay. I hear the kind of things you say when you fight. But people don't end marriages of 20 years because one partner gets angry easily or because they don't have good communication with the children. Something has been going on that has built up over time. There have been two separations, and Donna is again asking you to leave, so I have to assume there is a serious problem. You can try to ignore it and hope it goes away or you can try to understand and resolve what is wrong.

I: I just can't understand what's going on with her. She keeps telling me to leave. I'm not doing anything wrong. I don't want to leave. I don't like living in a little two bedroom apartment. I've worked hard all my life. We are financially set. Now we are in a place where we could be comfortable, travel, start living.

The only thing I can figure out is that she's got a boyfriend. Is that it, Donna? You have someone else and want me out?

challenging those that may upset her. Ivan is aware of his bellicose behavior but does not think of it as inappropriate, as the people around him do not let him know it is inappropriate.

Ivan denies his part of the difficulty and returns to the basic problem as he sees it—the need for their marriage to remain intact.

Donna projects onto the children her own feelings about the relationship.

I interrupt their established way of communicating; their complain-defend process. After pointing out what they already know, that this is a serious problem between them that is eating away at their relationship and needs some attention now, I attempt to focus on their responsibility and choices for future work. Donna's feelings make no sense to Ivan. He does not really want to know more about what goes on with her. He is more clear about his own needs, where he is and what he wants for the future. From Ivan's past experience in this marriage, Donna has always functioned as a selfobject whose role in life was to meet his needs. Despite 20 years together, he knows very little about her inner needs and feelings. He has experienced her as an extension of his own self. Since he doesn't know her well, he tries to guess what could be motivating her to act in ways that are ruining his plans.

D: I don't have anyone else. Not yet. But if I leave, there is hope. Maybe, I can find someone who will care for me and treat me like I'm somebody. Maybe I can become somebody. I'm nobody with you.

I: (almost shouting) You've got someone already. That's what it is.

D: I said I don't but I wish I did.

I: (to therapist) Maybe you can get the truth from her. She doesn't tell me anything.

T: It is hard for you to understand what is going on here. You are hoping to push Donna into telling you something that will make sense out of her behavior toward you.

I: Donna never talks to me. She never tells me anything. The only way I get anything out of her is when I get her to be angry. Then she tells me the truth.

T: So to get some communication you have to provoke her into an angry loss of control. Donna, do you recognize what Ivan is saying as happening often when you talk? That he needs to make you angry to get you to really talk to him.

D: That's why I hate to talk to him. He pushes me and pushes me until I do what he wants.

T: So the way Ivan attempts to communicate with you is what makes you want to avoid talking to him. What would happen if you tried telling him what is going on with you?

D: He doesn't listen. He already knows everything.

T: Ivan, do you think if Donna tries to sort out what is making her so upset with the relationship, you would be able to listen?

Donna reiterates the issue that is central for her at this point: the need to be separate, differentiated from her role as wife and mother, a caretaker for others rather than a person in her own right. She feels nonexistent and wants someone to make her feel good.

Ivan finds it difficult to understand what Donna needs. He thinks he knows what might be wrong. Ivan angrily tries to provoke Donna. He then turns to me in frustration.

I comment on his confused distress over her actions toward him and his attempt to control her, to get her to say something that will clarify the situation and help him know what to do.

Ivan explains how he provokes Donna to anger in order to reduce his own confusion and frustration.

I address my comments to both of them. This is part of an interactional pattern that can cause ongoing fights. He is upset and angry. She withdraws—he provokes her anger. When she is angry, he gets her back. But not as he wishes. She responds, but in a demanding, confrontational way rather than as the soothing selfobject that he is searching for.

I focus on their communication process to examine more about what doesn't work, and to see if there is a way to change the interactional pattern somewhat.

After identifying a pattern of communication between Ivan and Donna that causes problems, I try to help them to consider alternative

I: Sure. Tell me.

T: Donna, do you believe him?

D: No.

T: Shall we try and see what happens? I will attempt to clarify what you are saying so that Ivan will understand.

D: Last year, I suddenly realized that there was no "me" in this relationship. Everybody is so busy with you, "the great Ivan." I'm just sitting there with nothing to do. The kids don't need me very much. You don't need me. I've got to find out who I am and find something for myself.

I: What do you mean, I don't need you. Of course, I need you. You're my wife.

D: For what? Last year while you were on location in Canada, you called me and asked me to come. I came. When I got there, you didn't even talk to me. You were busy with all your important work.

I: We were shooting a scene. There was no time. What did you get so mad about? You know my work schedule when we are shooting.

D: What did you invite me for?

I: I wanted you to see what we were doing. It was the best part of the picture.

T: You wanted Donna to see what you had accomplished and when you first called her, didn't think that you might become too busy with work to see much of her. Meanwhile, she was feeling ignored and unimportant. Neither of you got what you wanted.

D: Then when we flew home, the stewardess kept making a big deal over you. "Are you comfortable, sir? Can I get you anything Mr.

ways of communicating with each other. I offer the possibility that something can be different this time.

If partners have a reservoir of good will and a willingness to try something different, a small change may lead to new patterns of operating together. When partners are narcissistically vulnerable and feel deeply hurt by each other, changes lead to defenses and new resistances. In such cases, a deeper level of work may be necessary. I begin with the least complex way of changing behavior. When this does not result in change, I go on to work with the narcissistic vulnerability and defenses.

Donna tries to explain the narcissistic injury that made her angry enough to decide to change her life. It seems almost insignificant to Ivan.

I note his need for mirroring and her need for a separate identity. He desperately wants his wife to look at his work with an approving gleam in her eye. She is no longer willing to give it because she is not getting recognition from him or from others.

I provide a linking comment, showing the underlying feelings of disappointment of each. Donna is not only upset by the lack of attention that she received from her husband, but also envious of his fame. She hates the attention he gets and feels that recognition is taken away from her. She may even wish to spoil the good things she thinks he is getting with all the attention.

___?" Well, what about me? Shouldn't I be comfortable? Can't she get me anything? That's why I got so mad on the way home. With you, I am nobody. Well, I am somebody.

T: I see. You were becoming increasingly upset with Ivan and with the reactions everyone has to him, while they almost ignored you.

D: And I have a right to have the friends I choose without you telling me that they shouldn't be in the house.

I: You mean Saturday? I don't want them in my bedroom. I don't know those women, and I don't know what they were doing there.

D: It's my bedroom, too, and my dressing area—and my friends. And, I don't want you telling me who to see or what I can do in my house.

I: Okay, okay.

T: You are saying, Donna, that you need more than just being a wife and mother. It feels as though neither Ivan nor the children need so much of the nurturing and loving you always had to give.

You are trying to find a new place for yourself, something important for you, not just as an extension of others. Your own choice of friends. Activities that are up to you. You haven't felt that you could do it if you remain married to this well-known, successful man. You haven't been able to explain what you are trying to do to him because you think he won't listen to you. Perhaps he can if he comes to understand what it means to you. Ivan, up to now it must have been very confusing. All of a sudden Donna is acting different-

Donna turns to other complaints now that she thinks she will be heard. She is no longer the silent or withdrawn person that I saw at the beginning of the session. Instead, she is expressing the anger that she previously felt she must hold in.

I interrupt the argument between them to identify for each what appears to be causing the problem. I try to summarize some of the needs, hurts, and ways each defends against injuries in general and give them some focus for future work. As I am talking, I carefully watch the facial expressions and body movements of each for signs of agreement, disagreement or confusion in either of them.

After suggesting how Donna may defend against feelings of hurt and vulnerability, I turn to Ivan with

ly than she ever has. Donna always took care of things so you could put your energies into your work. You were trying to figure out the change with only the bare minimum of information. So you thought of possible answers. While you were trying to sort out what was going on, you were also telling Donna how important this relationship is to you. How you may leave when she tells you to but you keep working toward a reconciliation. Perhaps Donna hasn't been able to listen to how you feel. I think we have some important issues to deal with, and clearly you're both being here says that each of you wants to make it better. **D:** How long do you think we will have to come? I don't like the way some people go to analysts for years.

T: I think we should plan for 12 sessions and then evaluate where we are and where the two of you are together.
I: Fine.
T: This time next week will work for me. How about you?
  Both agree.

some understanding of how difficult and confusing Donna's new behavior must feel to him.

I present a nonjudgmental view of his attempt to make this relationship work and point out the value of both involving themselves in treatment.

This question alerts me to the possibilities of underlying fear and anxieties about the therapeutic process and about areas that Donna feels too vulnerable to touch. I note her concern about getting into treatment but respond to the surface level question, at this point. We have a goal and time limit to this treatment and a time when we will evaluate together. Therapy should feel less threatening at a later time.

CASE DISCUSSION

Life transitions often cause a crisis to partners who have stabilized a relationship in which each has performed a selfobject function for the other. Donna was a mirroring selfobject for Ivan, and his extraordinary successes made him an idealized selfobject for her. As they near fifty, and their children leave home, there is a transformation that is destroying the stable interactions that were carefully built up and precariously maintained. While there is considerable narcissistic vulnerability in each, the current problems of Donna and Ivan are not due to their pathologies so much as to their failure to function as good selfobjects for each other; as they did in the past.

As the sessions progressed, it became evident that both had experienced emotional failures in childhood and each had vulnerable areas. But for many years each was very careful to soothe, reassure and affirm the strong points of the other. Donna had many fears about her ability to function in the world. Ivan's constant reinforcement of her importance as a homemaker, wife, and mother made her feel valued and successful. It recreated her parents' reinforcement of what a "good girl" she was, "never giving us a moment of trouble."

She won love and approval for never developing a self of her own. Ivan was more rebellious as a child. He fought for autonomy but felt that he had to give up love and acceptance in exchange for becoming his own self. While he is quite certain that this enabled him to take the risks that made him successful, he finds himself still seeking approval from his parents, wife, and professional colleagues.

Just as his wife became upset because she felt unresponded to, he felt upset because she withdrew from him the affirmation he had come to expect. Once this began, the empathy that they both had for the needs of each other was used not to enrich but to damage the other. Until they began to listen to each other at the communication level of vulnerabilities and needs, they could not reestablish a nurturing relationship.

With a couple like Donna and Ivan, the choice was to deal with the immediate problems. As therapy progressed and they felt more secure, they began looking at some other issues and chose to continue treatment. We agreed to continue meeting for an additional twenty sessions, which we are doing currently. At a later time we will again evaluate to determine whether to proceed or to terminate.

SUMMARY

The goals of marital therapy depend on the couple, their degree of pathology, their fit, and their willingness and good will in participating in deeply held feelings for each other. A limited goal may be to help couples learn new ways of listening to each other and enhancing their ability to negotiate a comfortable relationship. A more depth-oriented focus is the recognition that interactional patterns are repetitions of early narcissistic injuries, and to learn how to translate what feels like demands or attacks into messages of needs and vulnerability.

At a deeper level, for those willing to invest considerable time and emotional energy into the relationship, partners can become selfobjects for each other, with an enhancement of the process of firming the formerly enfeebled self of each. Clearly this goal is achievable only with some couples seen in conjoint therapy. However, I have known and worked with couples whose marriages became the therapeutic relationship that resulted in revitalizing self-confidence and enthusiasm for achieving goals.

I have also treated couples whose very severe problems were contained for long periods of time as both felt their needs were being met by the other. As outside stresses increased the neediness and vulnerability of each and put pressure on the ability of each to provide for the needs of the other, the relationship began to deteriorate, and therapy was initiated. In such cases the work requires treatment of underlying individual issues in conjunction with repairing selfobject functions of each for the other.

REFERENCES

Bowen, M. (1972), On the differentiation of self. In: *Family Interaction: Dialogue Between Family Researchers and Family Therapists*, ed. J. Framo. New York: Springer.

Bowen, M. (1976), Theory in the practice of psychotherapy. In: *Family Therapy: Theory and Practice*, ed. P. J. Guerin. New York: Garner Press, pp. 42–91.

Dicks, H. (1967), In: *Marital Tensions*. New York: Basic Books.

Kohut, H. (1971), *The Analysis of the Self*. New York: International Universities Press.

_____ (1977), *The Restoration of the Self*. New York: International Universities Press.

_____ & Wolf, E. S. (1978), The disorders of the self and their treatment. *Internat. J. Psycho-Anal.*, 59:413–425.

Lang, J. (1985), Passionate attachments. Lectures at Passionate Attachments Seminar. Los Angeles, CA.

Solomon, M. (1985), Treatment of narcissistic and borderline disorders in marital therapy: suggestions toward an enhanced therapeutic approach. *Clin. Soc. Work Journal*, July: 141–156.

_____ (1988), *Narcissism and Intimacy*. New York: Norton.

Author Index

Subject Index